THE VITALITY DIET

The 1990s health plan: how to slim your way to health and
fitness with a balanced diet specially adapted to suit your
individual needs

THE VITALITY DIET

The revolutionary health plan
that can change your life

Dr Alan Stewart and Maryon Stewart

THORSONS PUBLISHING GROUP

First published 1990

British Library Cataloguing in
Publication Data

Stewart, Alan
  The vitality diet.
  1. Physical fitness. Slimming. Diet
  I. Title   II. Stewart, Maryon
  613.2'5

  ISBN 0-7225-2101-4

*Published by Thorsons Publishers
Limited, Wellingborough,
Northamptonshire NN8 2RQ, England*

Typeset by Harper Phototypesetters
Limited, Northampton, England
**Printed in Great Britain by
Mackays, Chatham, Kent**

10   9   8   7   6   5   4   3   2

Contents

Part Two

About the authors

Dr Alan Stewart is a doctor specializing in nutritional therapy and a founding member of the British Society for Nutritional Medicine, as well as medical adviser to the Women's Nutritional Advisory Service. Alan qualified in 1976 from Guy's Hospital, London, and is a member of the Royal College of Physicians.

Maryon Stewart runs the highly acclaimed Women's Nutritional Advisory Service, which was established in 1987 following the success of the PMT Advisory Service. Maryon studied preventive dentistry and nutrition at the Royal Dental Hospital in London.

The couple live in Sussex with their three children.

Acknowledgements

We would like to thank the many doctors and scientists in the United Kingdom and abroad who have been involved in research into nutrition and obesity. Their publications have been essential to the writing of this book.

Our sincere thanks go to all the patients who have volunteered to share their experiences and allowed us to divulge intimate details about them, in the hope of helping others.

We also thank the team of dedicated workers at the Women's Nutritional Advisory Service for their professionalism over the years, which has enabled us to collect much of the research material referred to in this book.

Special thanks are due to Sarah Tooley, Senior Nurse at the WNAS, for her contributions to the menus and recipes and for her total support; Rosa Fisher, for her ongoing support and optimism; and to Jane Booker, our wonderful Nanny, who kept our three children happy and occupied while we were burning the midnight oil.

Additionally, we would like to thank Debbie, Jenny P, Henrietta, Gina, Sue, Michelle, and Jenny T, for being so willing to work unusual hours, and maintaining their sense of humour, particularly at the eleventh hour when one word processor blew up and the other erased the text!

Finally, we would like to thank our three wonderful children, Phoebe, Chesney, and Hester, for their patience and understanding whilst we were preoccupied.

Maryon & Alan Stewart

Introduction

There have been many books written on diet in relation to weight loss, and therefore one may justifiably ask why there is a need for another book on the subject.

You have probably tried a variety of methods of losing weight with temporary success, only to find that the weight goes right back on again as soon as you return to your normal diet. Rapid weight loss may have made you feel good at the time, but depression and frustration soon set in as the pounds or kilos slowly creep back on again.

Sometimes, even on the strictest of diets, allowing only a few hundred calories per day, it seems impossible to shift even a small amount of weight per week. It is disheartening to come to terms with the fact that your metabolism has adjusted to such a small calorie intake, and as a result your weight is unlikely to change.

For years now, at the Women's Nutritional Advisory Service, we have been working with people who have needed to make dietary changes for the sake of their health. They may have been suffering with anything from stress-related migraines to pre-menstrual tension. We have noticed that, by making adjustments to their diet, not only did they overcome their symptoms, but those who were overweight very often lost weight without even trying. They did not have to suffer a very low-calorie diet

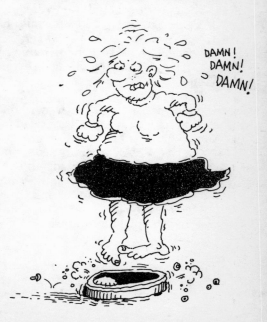

DAMN!
DAMN!
DAMN!

or one that involved eating expensive and unusual foods. Now doesn't that sound appealing?

We discovered that by making permanent changes to their usual diets individuals felt that their general health improved dramatically; they felt far better mentally, and they managed to lose those ugly pounds of flesh that had been slowing them down and stubbing their ego. It goes without saying that they were delighted with their progress and that their morale got an unexpected boost as a result.

Your individual needs

In order to lose weight permanently, and at the same time to rid yourself of some possibly long-standing unpleasant symptoms, you will need to learn what *your* body needs. We seem to know more about car maintenance

EILEEN RUFFELL

Eileen had a problem with her weight since the birth of her baby three and a half years ago.

'I was one and a half stones [21lb/9.5kg] overweight, I had awful headaches, desperate depression and chronic constipation.

'I had previously followed a diet in *Slimming* magazine and lost a stone and a half in weight. It was really hard going, so you can imagine how exasperated I felt when I put the weight back on again!

'I had felt very tired and irritable on the diet and was very depressed to see the weight going on again when I reverted to my previous eating habits.

'I lost 24lb [11kg] on the Women's Nutritional Advisory Service programme in two months without even trying to lose weight. I felt much better on the diet, I got rid of my constipation completely and even found that I had much more energy generally.

'On the WNAS programme I found that I had to stop eating wheat, in particular wholemeal bread, white bread and pasta. I did find it difficult to adjust to my diet at first, but I found that over a period of a few months my dietary habits changed and I got used to preparing different foods.

'I took regular supplements and exercised every day. I particularly enjoy walking and playing badminton. I have also joined a singing club. I have the energy to do all these things now that I am no longer tired and depressed.

'I feel so much better about myself. I have time for everyone. My family relationships are greatly improved as a result of my attitude and everyone says how happy and well I look now.'

than we do about our own bodies. We know that a car will come to a grinding halt if we put water in the petrol tank, so no one in their right mind does it! The same rule does not apply to our bodies, because we are not educated about what our individual bodies require in order to function optimally.

In the first part of this book we will be 'filling the education gap'. We will tell you all you need to know about surviving despite the twentieth-century diet, and the real facts about obesity. We will also help you to understand your own body so that you begin to know what your actual dietary requirements are. In Part Two of the book we will help you to work out a ten-week programme for you to follow. During the course of this programme you will learn how to become a 'nutritional detective', and put your new diet into practice. For each of the first eight weeks there is a weekly plan that will touch on a different aspect of your diet. By the end of this eight-week programme you will know about your body's requirements, and you should have managed to shake off those excess pounds. You will then know what a healthy weight-loss diet is for you and be able to follow this for a further two weeks, or longer if necessary.

Read each chapter in sequence and enjoy the knowledge. You should regard this as a nutritional adventure; one with lessons to last you a lifetime of good health, fitness, and slimness.

PART ONE

1
Filling the education gap

As children we are all taught how to read, write, and add up. Our parents teach us how to eat, dress, wash, and generally look after ourselves. But where and how do we learn about healthy eating? In general we are left to care for our own bodies, and those of younger members of the family. The woman is often regarded as the nutritional head of the household, and yet she has had little or no training for this job. For most other jobs that we take on in life, there will be an element of training, but, in the case of achieving or maintaining health through diet, this is not always so.

Let us give you some idea of just how important nutrition is. The major causes of death in developed countries are heart disease and cancer. Both are influenced to a large degree by the type of diet we eat. Up to 50 per cent of people with heart disease or cancer could probably have prevented or delayed the onset of their illness if they had eaten a better diet or stopped smoking. This is particularly important for those who become ill at a relatively young age; i.e. before 65 years. Furthermore, many minor ills are also influenced by diet. Problems such as migraine, high blood pressure, arthritis, kidney stones, premenstrual syndrome, eczema, insomnia and anxiety can all be caused by an unbalanced diet.

So learning about healthy eating and what is a healthy balanced diet for you is very important. At the Women's Nutritional Advisory Service we conducted a survey to find out what people understood by the term 'a balanced diet'. We also asked which foods contained key vitamins like C, B, A, D, and E, and some key minerals like magnesium, zinc and iron. The results of this survey would have been entertaining were it not for the fact that this is such a serious subject. The only information that people seemed to have about diet was the basic lesson from school, if they could remember it. Apart from knowing facts such as 'oranges contain vitamin C' and 'liver contains iron', hardly anyone had a clue as to what actually constitutes a sound balanced diet or even how much of each nutrient is required each day for their body size, or anyone else's body size for that matter.

In actual fact, there are some 15 vitamins, 24 minerals and 8-10 amino acids that have been isolated as being essential for normal body function. They are synergistic, which means they rely on each other in order to keep the body functioning at an optimum level. If you liken the body to a computer for a moment, the computer can only function when it has the correct data and commands fed to it; otherwise it refuses to work or breaks down altogether. Similarly, our bodies require the correct input of nutrients. When one or more nutrient is in short supply the body cannot function properly, and symptoms, be they physical or mental, occur.

'Ms AVERAGE'

A good example is one of a woman who went through her teenage years coping with the stresses of modern life and the hormonal changes that occurred in her body. She began to experience mild premenstrual tension, water retention and period pains. She also developed a sweet tooth, and occasionally had little chocolate binges. As time went on she settled into a busy, challenging job which she found both demanding and stressful. She lived alone, and therefore preferred convenience and fast foods rather than cook herself a proper meal with vegetables. She found that she gradually became prone to weight gain and as a result experimented with several different diets. She would go from eating little and missing meals to eating heavily at times when she experienced her sweet cravings.

Eventually, she married and had her first baby. She gained some 25lb (11kg) in weight during her pregnancy, half of which she lost whilst breast-feeding for six months. Her pre-menstrual tension became worse after the birth of her baby and she felt generally under par. A couple of years later she had her second baby and again breast-fed for a few months after the birth. She gained even more weight this time, which she had trouble shifting.

From that point on, her life became a juggling act. She had to look after the family and the home, and sometimes she even had a part-time job as well. She had little time to care for herself, and even less time for planning and preparing meals with proper thought and care. She was now 15lb (7kg) heavier than she had been in her single days; she felt tired and run down, and suffered with migraines, abdominal bloating, and increasing premenstrual symptoms including irritability, nervous tension, depression, tearfulness, confusion, weight gain, sore breasts, and insomnia. Worst of all, her self-image was low with the best years of her life fast disappearing, taking her previous good health with it and leaving her with the excess baggage. It would be the last straw if her husband tried to get romantic at the wrong time of the month.

A common tale but, we're sure you will agree, not a pretty picture. This woman was never taught how to cope with the stresses of modern living and how a good diet and lifestyle can help. Furthermore, she was not aware that the physical stress of pregnancy and breast-feeding all place greater nutritional demands on the body, which need to be met. Had she known more about healthy eating and what was right for her body, she might well have been able to prevent most of the problems that she experienced. If she had been feeling fitter and healthier, she certainly would have been better equipped to deal with the stresses, and to control her weight gain before it got out of hand.

Obviously, in a situation like this it is not only the woman herself who suffers. Her husband and her children can really be on the receiving end of her mood changes, and directly affected by her energy levels and her lack of knowledge about good nutrition. The quality of food she serves at home may influence not only her own health but also her children's growth and development, as well as her husband's cholesterol level.

All these unfortunate factors could have been avoided through good education and adequate nutrition. Part of our mission in this book is to 'fill the education gap' in many people's upbringing.

2
Twentieth-century diet

Obesity is an increasingly common problem, and there are many other serious conditions that have increased dramatically in recent years, the more serious of which, such as high blood pressure and heart disease, are associated with obesity.

In Britain alone it is estimated that in excess of 150,000 people die every year from heart attacks and strokes. In the United States it is reported that some 35 million Americans now suffer with high blood pressure, and one and a half million heart attacks and strokes occur each year.

Problems like premenstrual tension, and hyperactivity in children are on the increase, as well as a number of conditions that are caused by allergies of one kind or another: hay fever, eczema, asthma, migraine, and even some bowel problems.

You may well ask why we seem to be becoming a sick and overweight society. The fact is that our twentieth-century diet and lifestyle brings us new experiences that we are not well equipped to deal with. The diet and lifestyle that are common to many of us are far removed from those of our ancestors.

FACTS ABOUT TWENTIETH-CENTURY DIET

Sugar

We have vastly increased our consumption of sugar, averaging some 80 pounds (36kg) of sugar per person per year.

Animal fat

Our diets are too high in animal fats, also known as saturated fats, which contribute greatly to obesity and heart disease, and are associated with breast cancer.

Tea and coffee

We are high consumers of tea and coffee, both of which block the absorption of many essential nutrients and can aggravate anxiety and insomnia.

Salt

We eat 10–20 times more salt than our bodies actually require. This can cause a small rise in blood pressure and promotes water retention. It needs to be avoided by those who have these problems.

Junk food

Processed and pre-prepared foods have become a tempting and convenient option in recent times. They are designed to be quick to prepare and even quicker to eat and as a result are highly desirable to anyone who has a busy lifestyle. The processing of such food greatly reduces its normal vitamin content. For example, McDonald's apple pie (presumably made with apples) when analysed contained no vitamin C, when according to standard food values it should contain several milligrams. The famous 'Big Mac' has only a fraction of the vitamin B content it should have. You would have to eat 60 a day in the UK to get your full intake of vitamin B if this was your only source of food. The Big Macs in the USA contain 6 times as much vitamin B_6 as those in the UK.

Additives

Many of the foods available to us contain chemical additives in the form of colourings, stabilizers, flavour enhancers and preservatives. While some of these are not harmful, the full effects of many of them are unknown. Our bodies were certainly not designed to cope with them and some people can be sensitive to them, producing a variety of allergies.

Meat

The meat we consume is often too fatty. Good quality, additive-free, fresh lean meat is an excellent food, but our fast food philosophy means we may eat a lesser version.

Drinking water

It is accepted now that drinking water in many areas contains certain pollutants which are undesirable. The quality of drinking water in some parts of the UK does not satisfy the World Health Organization guidelines, particularly with regard to levels of lead and nitrates. Both are toxic. Though the levels are still low, it is their slow accumulation that appears to be important. Lead may affect child development and nitrates increase the cancer risk.

Social poisons

As well as the dietary factors there are the 'social' substances that many of us know and love. Sadly these also affect our nutritional state and health. These include alcohol, tobacco, drugs, and even tea and coffee. Amazingly, for every £1 spent on food in the UK in 1985, 76 pence was spent on alcohol and tobacco.

Drugs

Western societies have become drug orientated. In the USA in 1984 over one billion dollars was spent on drugs. In the UK for the same period

£1,600 million was spent on drugs, 50 per cent more than was spent in 1980. In the UK alone, over £40 million per year is spent on tranquillizers, and it is estimated that at least 3 million people are addicted to them. Some drugs affect appetite and also increase the need for vitamins and minerals. This particularly affects the elderly, those on long-term drugs for epilepsy, and those taking water pills for heart disease and high blood pressure.

What does all this mean? These are all the potential problems we are exposed to in the twentieth century. The news is by no means all bad; quite the opposite. In practice we now have a greater quantity of food, more choice of different foods with less seasonal variation and of better quality than ever before, all at a cheaper price. Consequently, we have, in fact, been able to eat a better diet this century, and this — com-bined with improvement in housing, immunization and some modern drugs — has meant a greatly improved standard of health and life expectancy. In the main, the biggest improvements have been in child health and the process of childbirth.

The point is that we have a choice; in fact, a great variety of foods to choose from — many good, some bad. In order to make the right choices we need two things: some reliable facts to educate ourselves with, and some experience of how different foods affect the body, our own in particular. So, in Part One we are giving you the education, and in Part Two we will introduce you to some carefully designed experiments, as well as some more education so you can become your own diet and weight-loss expert. You can more than survive the twentieth-century diet; you can flourish on it if you know how to make the right choices.

3
Fat chance — where other diets go wrong

Somehow we are sure that this is not the first diet book you have ever bought, or indeed the first time you have tried to lose weight. If you have tried any other diets, it might help to know something about some of the most recent and popular ones. Many previous, and indeed popular, diets have been based upon fads and fashions and not as scientifically based as they might be. All these diets are low-calorie ones, and for many people they have been highly successful. Any low-calorie diet will work, if adhered to. What determines their long-term success is whether they suit your metabolism or not. If a diet contains foods that you find hard to digest, or react to, then quite simply you are not going to stick to it.

So let's look at some diets. **The Scarsdale Medical Diet** was developed by Dr Tarnower, a family doctor from New York. His diet was a very high protein, low carbohydrate diet. The disadvantage is that it was very expensive, low in fibre, and not well balanced for use in the long term. It was probably most useful as a crash diet for two or three weeks.

The Beverly Hills Diet, by Mazel and Schultz, was a good example of one of the fad diets emanating from the USA. The diet was mainly based upon fruit, and was thus high in fibre but extremely low in protein, and poorly balanced for nutrient intake. It could only be followed for a limited period of time. Living off paw-paw (papaya), mango and pineapple might sound delicious, but is not practical for the long term.

The 'F' Plan Diet, originated in the UK by Audrey Eyton, is one of the most successful diet books in recent years. Quite rightly the stress was on fibre, but to the point that each day was yet another round of bran, wholemeal bread, and baked beans. If you could digest it, it was excellent, but many women found its side-effects intolerable. For them, the 'F' stood not for fibre, but for flatulence. We now also know that high intakes of bran may have a variety of adverse effects on nutritional balance, and in general vegetable and fruit fibre is a better bet.

Calorie-counting is used by professional dietary advisers, including hospital-based dietitians and weight-watchers. It is probably the best method for long-term weight control, since it educates you as to the calorie content and nutritional value of different foods. For the seriously overweight, we think that this is the best long-term method. However, like all the other diets listed, it takes no account of individual variations in ability to tolerate certain foods. Ideally, you want a diet that not only helps you to shed pounds in weight, but really makes you healthy, and the best way to do that is by finding out which foods suit you. If you have genuine difficulty in keeping to the diet in this book or any other diet, your best bet is to go back to the calorie-counting method, supervised by a diet club, dietitian, or doctor.

The Hip and Thigh Diet, a recent book by Rosemary Conley, recommends a diet and series of exercises to help lose weight, particularly from the hips and thighs. The principle is highly attractive. This is a high-fibre, well-balanced diet, but allows substantial quantities of dairy products and bread, which your body may not be able to tolerate. Furthermore, there is a fundamental fallacy. Fat deposition in the areas of hips and thighs is mainly related to the female hormone, oestrogen. Women naturally have larger bottoms and smaller waists than men, whose male hormone testosterone leads mainly to weight gain around the abdomen. There is no particular food that you need to avoid in order to help lose weight from the hips and thighs. The best way to

improve your shape is by exercise, of course.

The BBC Diet, as you would expect with this sort of title, is a very reliable sound diet that is recommended. Again, there is nothing wrong with it except that it is 'do as I say' and not 'let's find out what is right for you'. If it works and you felt great on it — then do it again.

Finally, if you had tried one or more of the above diets with lasting success, you wouldn't be reading this book! What we are going to do is find a diet that not only helps you to achieve effective weight loss, but is really healthy, suits your individual needs, and can be followed for years to come in order to maintain the weight and shape you want.

WHY DO FAT PEOPLE KEEP HAVING TO DIET?

Many weight-loss diets are successful in the short term but fail to keep the weight off long-term. However, if you have a car tyre that has a slow puncture, and you have to take it to the garage every week to put air into it, it doesn't mean that there is anything wrong with the pump: there must be something else wrong to make the tyre lose air. Likewise, there must be factors other than the diets themselves that cause them to fail. The tyre has a 'fault' and so, very often, has the overweight person. In the past it has been thought that the fault was greed, but this is too simple a view. The fault often lies within the body and with the person's perception of good health.

In short the healthier you become — by eating healthily, and choosing the foods that suit you — the more likely you are to eat healthily and maintain your correct weight in the long term. Eating badly and gaining weight is an unpleasant experience, and should be so different from your new lifestyle that you never want to do it again.

4
A diet to make you sick

You may feel that we have been exaggerating about the goodies we like to consume causing us shape and health problems. There is, however, no getting away from the truth that alcohol, cigarettes, sugar, tea and coffee do interfere with the balance of nutrients in the body.

THE EXPERIMENT

The idea was to take a person who was in excellent nutritional shape and consuming a good, better than average diet without taking any vitamin or mineral supplements, who was a non-smoker and moderate consumer of alcohol, sugar, tea, coffee and chocolate; and to see what effect consuming the national average amount of alcohol, cigarettes, sugar, tea, coffee and chocolate would do to this fine healthy specimen.

As Maryon had not long had a baby, we decided that Alan should volunteer, as he did not have such a valid excuse! So he became our guinea pig.

Two weeks before the experiment began, Alan's blood levels of vitamins and minerals were measured. They were measured again at the start of the experiment and every two weeks during the 'active' phase which was due to last for eight weeks.

As well as his usual diet, Alan had to consume the following each day:-

tea	4 cups per day
coffee	2 cups per day
alcohol	3 units per day (1 unit = 1 glass of wine, 1 measure spirit or half a pint of beer or lager)
chocolate	1 small chocolate bar per day (approximately half a large Mars Bar)
soft drinks	½ can of cola
sugar	12 teaspoons per day, i.e. two teaspoons in each of the hot drinks
cigarettes	6 per day.

The tea was made according to the instructions given by the Tea Council in London — brewing the tea bag for three minutes then squeezing it. The cigarettes were smoked properly, with each being inhaled as much as possible.

The first week

Maryon felt quite apprehensive about this experiment and wondered what it would be like to live with Alan during the diet. She also had some concern as to whether in eight weeks Alan might develop a taste for the alcohol, the chocolate, and even the cigarettes!

The first few days were very trying for Alan as he went on to the new regime suddenly rather than gradually. He had previously drunk hardly any tea, one or two cups of coffee without sugar per day, had the occasional alcoholic drink, and smoked only the occasional cigar. He developed a quite severe migraine headache and felt very sick by Day 3 and he was on the verge of giving up. However, as he had made a start, he was determined to continue come what may . . .

The second week

During the second week Alan felt very run down. He developed a flu-like cold which lasted for several days. This again was most unusual, as he is rarely ill. He found that he was so full-up from all the liquid in his diet that he hardly had room for his evening meal. His usual hearty appetite for three courses was reduced to the point where he was pushing his main course around his plate complaining that he felt nauseated and tired.

The calories provided by the extra alcohol, sugar, and chocolate were some 500 to 600 per day, and as Alan did not gain weight during the experi-ment we know that his intake of good foods must have fallen by this amount, some 25 per cent of his normal daily intake.

The third week

Alan is usually a very even-tempered individual who has endless energy. He is often perky until at least midnight. By Week 3 he was nodding off to sleep in an armchair as soon as he had finished dinner. By 8.30 pm he was unconscious, and could not be roused. He also developed a slightly more aggressive attitude, and became a bit short-tempered at times. He was still feeling the nausea, especially after smoking. Constipation was becoming a problem. He just couldn't eat the amount of fruit and vegetables he had tucked into before. Also, the tea and coffee with two teaspoons of sugar in each were not helping. By the time he had drunk them, mainly in the morning, his stomach was rumbling and churning like a cement mixer.

The fourth week

By Week 4 Alan's libido began to wane. His usual enthusiasm had definitely disappeared; more often than not he was unconscious anyway. By this time our former lifestyle was fast becoming a memory.

The fifth week

We wondered during the fifth week how Alan was going to manage to

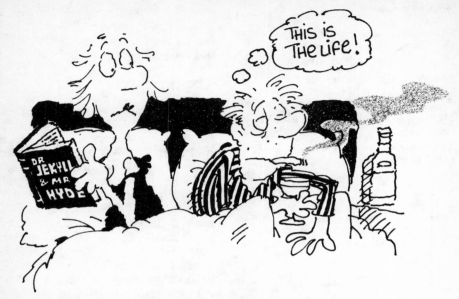

keep going for another four weeks. Maryon was getting a bit worried about him after an evening out in a restaurant: he had been getting behind with his alcohol intake so he decided to catch up. He consumed a bottle of Frascati and smoked two cigarettes, then turned green, almost passed out, and fell asleep sitting up in the chair.

Although the Laboratory was not meant to divulge any results to Alan until the eight-week period was over, it was decided that it might be better to know the results at six weeks, and perhaps to end the experimental diet at this point. Alan and Maryon both felt that six weeks would probably be enough and did not think he could manage to continue on this diet for another three weeks.

The sixth week

By the sixth week Alan was feeling pretty ill. He was very tired and found it hard to concentrate for long periods of time. One lunchtime, after consuming his ration of junk food and two cigarettes, he fell asleep on a sofa in his waiting room with a can of cola in his hands. When his first patient of the afternoon arrived before he awoke he knew it was time to abandon the diet. Fortunately, the patient saw the funny side of the situation!

By that time we both knew that enough was enough. The smoking, the drinking and the sugar were obviously not for Alan so we ended the experiment there.

LABORATORY RESULTS

It was just as well that Alan did decide to complete the diet after six weeks, as it turned out that many of his vitamin and mineral levels were sinking very fast.

Vitamin A

Alan's vitamin A levels fell by nearly 50 per cent in six weeks. Vegetable vitamin A, carotene, fell by 30 per cent, and both were now at the lower end of the normal range. Vitamin A is necessary for healthy vision and resistance to infection, and a good intake reduces the risk of cancer.

Vitamin A deficiency usually only occurs in the presence of a grossly inadequate diet or when severe digestive problems exist.

Vitamin B group

Vitamins B_1 (thiamin), B_2 (riboflavin) and B_6 (pyridoxine) were measured. From their healthy normal levels at the start, mild deficiencies of all three developed after six weeks. B-group vitamins are necessary for protein and energy metabolism. Deficiency can affect mood, energy level, skin quality, and resistance to infection.

Vitamin C

Alan's vitamin C levels fell rather dramatically, from the top end to almost the bottom end of the normal range by the end of the six week experimental diet. This level was by no means low enough to cause scurvy as Alan was still eating fruit and vegetables, though less than before. Interestingly, the first symptom of vitamin C deficiency is depression. Smokers are known to have lower vitamin C levels than non-smokers. It was probably this that affected Alan's vitamin C level the most.

Vitamin E

Alan's vitamin E level also fell by some 30 per cent from the middle to towards the bottom of the normal range. The vitamin E level would have had to fall much further to produce a deficiency and this would have been unlikely to happen in Alan or anyone else unless they are eating a very poor diet indeed.

Zinc

This important mineral also fell slightly by some 15 per cent. No deficiency developed, which is just as well because zinc has important functions influencing sex hormone and sperm production, resistance to infection, and appetite.

Magnesium

This fell by 10 per cent. Again, no deficiency developed and this fall was almost certainly caused by the reduced intake of green vegetables, a major source of magnesium, and the increased losses from the body that can occur with alcohol and coffee consumption. Magnesium is needed for the energy-producing steps in normal metabolism.

Chromium

The blood level of this mineral also fell from a very good healthy level to the lower end of the normal range. Chromium helps to control blood sugar and cholesterol levels in the body. A high sugar intake, which was part of Alan's diet, greatly increases the loss of chromium in the urine. It is thought that high sugar intakes and low chromium levels predispose to hardening of the arteries and raised cholesterol levels in later life.

Selenium

This mineral dropped by 15 per cent during the six weeks. This small fall did not produce a deficiency which anyway is rare in the well-fed normal population. However, those who have lower levels of selenium may have an increased risk of cancer in later years. The same seems to be true of vitamins A and E. The best food sources of selenium are fish and whole grains.

Other minerals

Levels of calcium, iron, copper, and manganese were also measured without any fall being evident.

Well, what does all this mean? Certainly, the average consumption of alcohol, cigarettes, sugar, and possibly even tea, coffee and chocolate do not help our nutrition

balance. People will vary enormously as to how their bodies tolerate these dietary items and you will learn in Stage II of the diet how your body gets on with some of these.

After the end of the sixth week Alan stopped the cigarettes, sugar and tea, and the extra coffee, alcohol and chocolate. Within three days he felt that he had been born again. Only then did he fully realize that he had been experiencing a mild dull pressure in the head, as well as the nausea, physical and mental fatigue.

For the next eight weeks, Alan went back to his old diet — again not taking any supplements. Within that time, all the vitamin and mineral levels were restored and Alan once again enjoyed good health apart from another cold, two weeks after stopping smoking and drinking.

CONCLUSION

What does this rather unusual experiment mean? Firstly, it is difficult if not dangerous to argue that what happens in one case happens in all. It does not. Some can smoke heavily, drink significant amounts of alcohol and get away with it. We know that it is easier for your body to tolerate the habit if you also eat well but many do not. Others feel ill at just the smell of cigarette smoke or even a glass of wine.

We are all different: but, certainly it is possible that for many of us our current consumption of cigarettes, alcohol, tea, coffee, sugar, and even chocolate are enough to adversely affect our health and our nutritional balance. Even the average consumption of these can be harmful for us. For many of us, reducing our consumption or even stopping all of them for a while is likely to help us in a number of ways. For example, on average some 25 per cent of calorie intake is derived from alcohol and sugar. As they are very poor quality foods they really form no part of a weight-reducing diet. Consumed in small quantities as part of a healthy diet (once your weight is normal), they probably do no harm and their pleasures are of course well known. More details about alcohol, sugar, tea, coffee, chocolate, and cigarettes are given in Part Two.

So we have seen how ill the average consumption of these can make one person feel. We will see, in Part Two, how much better stopping them could make you feel. Remember, we want you not only to lose weight but to feel really healthy with your body in good nutritional balance.

5
Understanding obesity

In developed countries, obesity is now probably the most common diet-related disorder. In developing countries, obesity is usually a mark of prosperity. Being overweight may be a distinct advantage in a country or community that is used to food shortages. Those who are thin and lean may fare less well than their plump counterparts at times of shortage. Unfortunately, we cannot use such excuses for ourselves, and so let's get down to some hard facts; facts which we think will give you an understanding of why you are overweight, and how this can best be tackled, in the short and long term.

First of all, how do we define obesity? On this page you will see a graph which gives measurements for height and weight. The graph is divided up into five sections, −1, 0, 1, 2, and 3. These are grades of weight, based on weight and height, from a formula originally derived from a Belgian scientist, Quetelet. He developed an index known as Quetelet's Index, which is widely used in the assessment of obesity. The categories are as follows:

−1: less than 20
 0: 20-25
 1: 25-30
 2: 30-40
 3: greater than 40

Normal or ideal weight is grade 0. Grade 1 is overweight, usually between 10 and 20 per cent above the ideal weight; grades 2 and 3 are

Height/weight chart showing the Quetelet grades of obesity

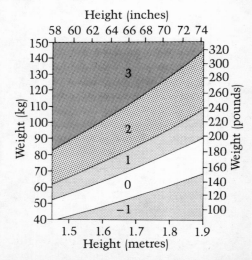

regarded as obese — more than 20 per cent above the ideal weight.

As measured by Quetelet's Index, the range associated with the greatest life expectancy and lowest death-rate is 20–25. There is a very slight rise in death-rate in those who are mildly overweight, grade 1, and also in those who are underweight, grade −1. But this low rise is so small as to be insignificant. It is grade 2, and especially grade 3, obesity, which carry the greatest risk to health. An individual with a Quetelet's Index of 40 has three times the risk of dying in a year than someone whose weight is ideal. An individual with a Quetelet's Index of 35 has approximately twice the death rate of his or her or her ideal counterpart.

In the UK, it is estimated that 1 in 4 people are overweight to some degree. For the majority who are just slightly overweight, grade 1 obesity, the major reasons for dieting are cosmetic and a sense of well-being. Not being overweight, and having a slim, attractive shape, is by current fashion highly desirable. Many of us will feel better psychologically when that spare tyre has been slimmed away, and if the diet is combined with an exercise programme there can be a very real improvement in feelings of overall fitness. Medically there is little change in factors such as blood pressure, and risk of heart disease, though there could be a moderate fall in blood cholesterol level if this is elevated at the start of the diet.

For those with grade 2 or 3 obesity, the potential benefits of losing weight are very real, and the effects on psychological state of a successful weight-loss programme can be dramatic. For example, normal employment is very difficult for those who are grossly overweight, grade 3 obesity.

THE HEALTH RISKS OF OBESITY

The obese, grades 2 and 3, especially the young, have a shorter life expectancy, and an increased risk of many illnesses, including diabetes, high blood pressure, heart disease, osteoarthritis, gout, gallstones, reduction in exercise tolerance/level of fitness, and depression.

Furthermore, general medical problems may be more difficult to care for in those who are obese. Gastro-intestinal disorders including indigestion, heartburn, and constipation, may be more difficult to assess in an obese individual, as the information obtained from a medical examination may be limited. Additionally, the survival rate of the obese woman with breast cancer is less than her thin counterpart.

The young obese individual who loses weight to normal or near-normal value may have a substantial improvement in life quality and expectancy, and reduction in risk in practically all of the above. The improvement in arthritis, gout, blood pressure, diabetes, or blood cholesterol level may be dramatic, and evident within a few weeks or months of a dietary programme.

WHAT CAUSES OBESITY?

Genetic factors

Analysis of families shows that if both parents are obese, 70 per cent of the children will also be obese. If one parent is obese, 40 per cent of the children will be obese, and if both parents are lean, then only 10 per cent will be obese. Clearly, the predisposition of the parents is carried down partially to the children. Of course, we could argue that obese parents eat too much, and are thus likely to overfeed their children, making them obese, and that it has nothing to do with genetics or inheritance. However, in studies of children who have been adopted, the adopted children take after the weight characteristics of their biological parents, rather than after their adopted parents. This and other work lends substantial support to the idea that a tendency to obesity is to a large degree genetic.

If this was the only causative factor, there would be little that we could do about it, but there is another side to the coin.

Environmental factors

By environment is meant all the factors that occur around us and potentially influence our internal metabolism, which we have already seen is initially determined by genetic make-up. With regard to obesity, the most important environmental factors are the food supply, level of exercise, lifestyle, and social pressures.

If the food supply, for example, is so meagre that there is barely enough food to go round, or starvation conditions exist, then obesity will obviously disappear from the community at large. In such a situation, with a limited food supply, environment is more important than any genetic factor. However, when there is an abundance of food, this allows the obesity tendency to express itself fully. When food is plentiful, some 25 per cent of the population may become obese. This is practically the situation in the UK, and has been fully achieved in the most prosperous countries in the world, notably the USA.

The majority of obese individuals will have one parent who is overweight, and only a minority would be the offspring of two obese or two thin parents. At this point you might feel like going out to shoot your mother and father, and they in turn would feel like shooting their parents, but this isn't a very practical solution! Further impractical solutions include forbidding the obese to reproduce: the effect of this would be surprisingly small, and it would take several generations of extremely unpopular enforced birth control to even halve the rate of obesity in the population. Another equally undesirable solution is to restrict the food supply to the whole population, punishing lean and obese alike. Again, this is unlikely to win any favour with the population at large.

The only practical solution is in some way to limit the calorie intake of those who are overweight, while taking other steps to improve their rate of weight loss.

In conclusion, it does seem that some people were born to be fat, but are only able to be fat because of the relatively affluent society in which they live.

In the next chapter we will learn what factors control appetite and metabolism, and how we can use this to build a successful weight-loss programme.

6
Obesity — your questions answered

WHAT CAUSES OBESITY?

Quite simply, having a calorie intake greater than your needs causes obesity.

WHAT ARE METABOLISM AND METABOLIC RATE?

Metabolism is the series of chemical reactions that occur in each cell and each organ to keep the body running properly.

DO FAT PEOPLE HAVE A SLOW RATE OF METABOLISM?

No. The metabolic rate, i.e. the rate at which calories are burnt, is the same in obese individuals as it is in those of normal weight. At times it can be higher. The metabolic rate is mainly determined, not by body weight, but by the amount of muscle and other lean tissue in the body. Obese subjects have a slightly greater muscle mass than thin subjects, as they have to do extra work carrying the weight of their fat stores.

DOES METABOLIC RATE VARY WITH AGE?

Yes, as you get older, there is a slight decrease in metabolic rate, but this effect is very small.

DOES METABOLIC RATE VARY FROM PERSON TO PERSON?

Yes, people of the same age and build may have a difference in metabolic rate of up to one-third. That means some people may require one-third fewer calories than others, depending upon their metabolic type.

WHY IS IT EASIER TO LOSE WEIGHT IN THE FIRST WEEK OR TWO?

In the first weeks of a diet (up to four), half the weight loss is fat, and half water, as a result of changes in sugar and protein metabolism. This makes it easier to lose weight in the first few weeks, at a rate which can be up to 4lb per week. Thereafter, the weight loss slows down to approximately 1–2lb per week, depending upon the type of diet.

DOES MY METABOLIC RATE VARY WHEN I DIET?

Yes, the metabolic rate can reduce by 10 per cent during a calorie-restricted diet. The amount of fall in metabolic rate may vary considerably from person to person, just as metabolic rate varies from person to person. Some find losing weight easy and some difficult.

HOW LONG WILL IT TAKE ME TO REACH MY IDEAL WEIGHT?

If you have grade 1 obesity, it may take between six weeks and six months; grade 2 obesity, three to eighteen months; and grade 3 obesity, one to three years, depending upon your starting weight and how closely you adhere to a weight-loss programme. This assumes that the diet you are going to follow is reduced by 500 to 1,000 calories per day, which will then have to be derived from your body's fat store.

DOES MENTAL EXERCISE OR STRESS BURN UP CALORIES?

As a rule, no. Mental exercise, including reading this book, will not help you to burn up any extra calories. Stress, by stimulating certain hormones, may produce a small increase in metabolic rate, but this is not yet certain. Worrying about your weight is more likely to lead to comforting yourself with a piece of chocolate than it is to assist in burning up any calories.

HOW HEALTHY ARE CRASH DIETS?

Any severely restricted diet, particularly one providing in the region of 400 calories a day, can be highly successful, particularly in the short term. However, if weight loss is excessive, then muscle tissue rather than fat tissue is lost, and this in turn will slow down the metabolic rate, making it more difficult to lose weight thereafter.

WILL I HAVE TO DIET FOR EVER?

In one sense, yes; the diet which has resulted in excessive weight gain or inability to lose weight is not the diet that you need to eat in the future. In this sense, you need to change your diet and will be 'on a diet for ever'. It all depends on what you consider to be a normal healthy diet. The vast majority of obese people have been eating a normal *un*healthy diet, and changing is a matter of education and attitude as well as trial and error. That's what this diet is all about.

HOW CAN I TELL HOW MANY CALORIES ARE IN A MEAL?

In carefully conducted experiments,

neither fat nor normal-weight subjects have been particularly good at estimating the calorie content of a meal. Only reading and learning about nutrition and the nutrient values of food will help you. In this respect, you have to become your own nutritionist.

WHAT STOPS NORMAL-WEIGHT PEOPLE BECOMING FAT?

The precise factors that control an individual's body weight are not yet fully known. It does seem, however, that normal-weight people know when to stop eating, and fat people simply go on too long. A carefully constructed calorie-controlled diet, with eating plans and education, is a good way for you and your body to learn when to say no, and switch off the desire for food.

WHAT CONTROLS MY APPETITE?

There is a part of the brain called the hypothalamus, which contains an appetite control centre. A variety of factors seem to influence this part of the brain, including the sight, smell, and taste of food, as well as one's knowledge about healthy eating.

HOW CAN I INCREASE MY METABOLIC RATE?

The most consistent way to increase metabolic rate in both obese and normal-weight subjects is by physical exercise. Physical activity will maintain or increase the amount of muscle in the body and it is muscle that controls metabolic rate. Exercise raises the metabolic rate, not only at the time of activity, but also for a little while afterwards. In athletes, and Arctic explorers, there can be as much as a two-fold rise in metabolic rate, requiring the calorie intake to be doubled in order to maintain normal weight.

WHAT DOES MY BODY DO WITH THE CALORIES I EAT?

Four-fifths of the calories in the diet are required to maintain the normal energy production and metabolism of the body — just keeping the engine ticking over even if you are resting completely. We are aware of this calorie usage as production of heat by the body — in order to keep the body at 37°C, our normal temperature, a certain amount of energy is required, and this requires some 80 per cent of our calorie intake. Only 20 per cent is used in physical activity such as climbing stairs or carrying shopping.

COULDN'T I LOSE WEIGHT BY MAKING MY BODY NEED MORE CALORIES?

One could in theory increase calorie requirements by wearing fewer clothes, so that the body's metabolic rate has to increase in order to maintain a normal body temperature. While this is true in normal-weight subjects, it unfortunately is not true in the obese! Fat is an excellent insulator against the cold. If anything, the metabolism of the obese becomes more sluggish when exposed to cold. Perhaps this is why some overweight people feel the cold more than their normal-weight fellows.

IS FAT JUST A MEANS OF STORING CALORIES?

For the most part, fat is simply a store of calories, but there are specialized areas of fat, called brown fat, which are found in the back between the shoulder blades and around the area of the kidneys. In response to certain hormones, brown fat burns extra calories to generate heat. The type of diet we eat may influence the activity of brown fat, and thus our metabolic rate. However, this effect is small, but it may not be insignificant. Certain animals, and possibly some humans, show differences in the metabolism in their brown fat. Obese subjects have a slower rate of brown fat activity than those of normal weight. In this respect, they may truly have a lower metabolic rate.

DO HORMONES INFLUENCE OBESITY?

Very occasionally, serious hormonal problems may lead to obesity, but the vast majority of those who are overweight do not have any serious hormonal imbalance. However, hormonal levels may vary widely from person to person, just as metabolic rate may. Some hormones, such as insulin, are needed to control rises in the level of glucose in the blood. Obese people tend to have higher levels of insulin than those of normal weight, and the disadvantage of insulin is that it tends to further encourage the body to deposit rather than to burn up fat. This may start a vicious circle. Once you are fat, it is easier to lay down more fat. The only ways of breaking out of this vicious circle and reducing the levels of insulin are by losing weight, taking more exercise, and improving the quality of your diet.

In summary, the factors that control obesity are:

(1) calorie intake

(2) metabolic rate, which varies from person to person, and is mainly determined by the amount of muscles in the body

(3) exercise level, and how much this stimulates your body's rate of metabolism

(4) hormonal balance.

IS IT BETTER TO EAT ONE LARGE MEAL A DAY?

There seems to be little difference in the actual amount of weight lost whether you eat all your calorie allowance in one go, or spread it over the day. However, your body will lose more fat tissue and less muscle tissue if calorie intake is spread over three to five meals and snacks during the day. This is why we will be advising you to have three meals and one or two snacks per day. Nibbling, rather than gorging, is a healthier way to lose weight and a better way of satisfying your appetite.

Occasionally, hormonal disturbance, particularly of the thyroid gland, may lead to a slowing down or speeding up of the metabolic rate. Going on to a weight-reducing diet actually reduces the rates of hormone production by the thyroid, and in turn slows down the metabolic rate.

CAN I CHANGE MY METABOLIC RATE?

In brief, yes, you can, but it is going to take some doing.

Exercise

Firstly, the most powerful stimulus to metabolic rate is exercise. Physical exercise raises your metabolic rate, and if the exercise is prolonged and undertaken regularly, your metabolic rate will rise even at rest. Exercise does not necessarily have to be very vigorous, but it does need to be regular, and for a significant duration. The minimum amount would be three sessions of exercise per week, each lasting 30 minutes.

Protein intake

Secondly, ensuring a good intake of protein in the diet will help to minimize loss of muscle tissue during a weight-loss programme. Losing muscle tissue will slow down your metabolic rate, and this is just what you don't want. That's why we have devised a low-calorie, high-protein diet.

Intake of vitamins and minerals

Thirdly, certain vitamins and minerals may influence the production of thyroid hormones. Zinc and vitamin A, if deficient, may lead to a reduction in the output of hormones by the thyroid, and in turn a relative slowing of metabolic rate. While this is unlikely to be a problem in the early stages, being on a prolonged low-calorie diet which does not provide an adequate intake of these and other nutrients might have an adverse effect upon the body's metabolism, and make it increasingly difficult to either lose weight or to maintain your exercise level. This may well be a reason why previous diets have failed. Details about nutritional supplements to prevent this are on page 55.

Nutritional deficiencies

Finally, your level of physical activity is going to be influenced to a large degree by how well and how fit you feel. Muscles require substantial amounts of magnesium, potassium, vitamin B, protein, and zinc in order to work effectively. Severe deficiencies of these nutrients occur only rarely, but it is becoming increasingly appreciated that mild or borderline levels of these nutrients may be found not infrequently in the 'normal population'. Obese individuals, because of their less prudent eating habits, and/or differences in metabolism, may be at risk for mild deficiencies in these nutrients. Going on to a weight-reducing diet that is not adequately balanced may further compromise your feelings of well-being and energy, and limit the degree to which you can undertake an increased level of exercise. In the long run, this may have a significant effect upon your ability to control your own weight.

7
Getting the balance right

Now we are going to take a look at what it takes to keep a body healthy, and in particular at your nutritional requirements.

The two essential parts in looking at the adequacy of the diet are:

- whether the intake is adequate in amount
- whether the balance is correct.

Nowadays, lack of intake is not usually the problem, so we will turn our attention to balance.

The body could not survive healthily for very long on a diet composed of any one type of food. Not only would it be monotonous, it would also fail to provide the range of nutrients that the body requires for health. These are proteins, fats, carbohydrates, vitamins, minerals, and fluid.

ESSENTIAL NUTRIENTS

Proteins are the building-blocks of the body. Tissues, such as muscle, heart, liver, kidneys, and most other organs, are rich in protein. Skin, bones and hair also contain certain amounts of protein, which contributes to their structure. The main role of protein, however, is to perform the functions of each individual cell. Thus protein is necessary for the ovaries and thyroid to produce hormones, for the kidneys to make urine, for muscles to exercise, and so forth. If a large amount of protein is used in the diet, then some is used for energy purposes, and during starvation, protein is taken from the muscles of the body and used as a fuel supply. This tends to slow down the body's metabolic rate, and for this reason weight-loss diets should have plenty of protein. On average for every one stone (14 pounds/6.5kg) of body weight, we require a daily intake of some 5 grams of protein (about half an egg). This is essential to keep the body healthy.

Carbohydrates come in a variety of different forms, all of which are best regarded as sources of energy. The simplest forms of carbohydrate in our diet are glucose and fructose. These are single sugar units, and fructose is found particularly in high amounts in fruit; hence its name, which means fruit sugar. Fructose and glucose can be joined together to make sucrose or table sugar, normally prepared from sugar cane or sugar beet. Milk contains yet another type of sugar called lactose, which itself is composed of two single units of sugar: glucose and galactose.

So much for the simple carbohydrates. The complex carbohydrates, which are found in vegetables, cereals and to a lesser degree in fruits, are composed of numerous sugar units joined together in a complex way. These have to be broken down by the digestive system before they are absorbed as single units of mainly glucose and fructose.

Complex carbohydrates are desirable for three reasons:
- they are slowly digested and release their energy at a steadier rate
- foods rich in complex carbohydrates are also rich in vitamins and minerals, which are essential for the metabolism of sugar and the steady release of its energy
- such foods are also high in fibre, high intakes of which are associated with many health benefits.

Refined carbohydrates, such as sucrose and pure glucose, may be a convenient source of quick energy, but they lack vitamins, minerals, and fibre. They are all too easily

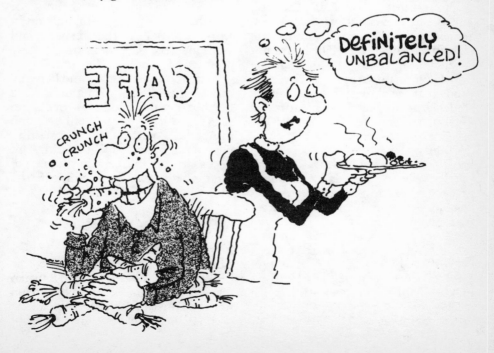

consumed to excess, and thus may lead to obesity.

Fats are a major source of energy in the diet, and provide twice as many calories as protein or carbohydrates for the same amount in weight. In developed countries, fat intake has increased at the expense of a reduction in complex carbohydrates. In order to lose weight, we almost always have to cut down on fat intake, but some fats are essential, just as vitamins and minerals are. These are the polyunsaturated fats, which are derived mainly from sunflower, safflower and rapeseed oils, vegetables, nuts, seeds and some fish.

Foods of animal origin, e.g. lard, dripping, butter, milk, cream, cheese, and meat, and some vegetable oils, notably palm oil and coconut oil, are rich in saturated fats. These are not essential, and have the undesirable effect of stimulating the liver to produce more cholesterol, and raising its level in the blood. Both saturated and polyunsaturated fats contain the same amount of calories.

Finally, cholesterol is a specialized form of fat which is found particularly in eggs, dairy products, and meat. Most of the cholesterol in our blood is actually made by our liver and approximately one-third is derived from our diet. Dietary cholesterol is not the ogre the experts once thought it was. Our dislike of late has turned quite rightly to an excess of animal fats, combined with a lack of fibre in the diet.

Approximately 15 per cent of our diet is composed of protein; 55 per cent is composed of carbohydrate, and 40 per cent of fat.

Vitamins and minerals are essential nutrients that are required not for their calorific value, which is negligible, but because they help regulate the body's metabolism. All vitamins and essential minerals are necessary to assist in normal functioning of the thousands of different chemical reactions that make up the body's metabolism. If the supply of vitamins and minerals in the diet is inadequate, this will result in changes in body chemistry, and a slowing down or altering of the body's metabolism, usually with some deterioration in body fitness or health. Vitamins and minerals often work together in this respect, and some are necessary for normal energy production, the use of protein in growth and tissue repair, and in many other functions, ranging from hormone production to effects on skin quality. Additionally, some minerals, particularly calcium, phosphorus and magnesium, are necessary with certain types of protein for the formation of the skeleton.

FIBRE

Fibre is a specialized form of complex carbohydrate, which cannot be broken down by the normal human digestive system. It thus becomes a major constituent of the waste product, faeces. Diets high in fibre are often high in vitamins and minerals, and a high-fibre diet is an important part of a weight-reduction programme — more of this in Chapter 9.

BALANCE

Part of a healthy weight loss programme is to get the nutritional balance right. On average, we have an adequate or slightly excessive intake of calories derived from fat and carbohydrate. Protein intakes are normally adequate, unless the diet is very restricted. The intake of vitamins and minerals is, if we are eating a healthy, well-balanced diet, almost certainly adequate, but how many of us are already eating a healthy, well-balanced diet?

At certain times of our lives, and in certain situations, it may be difficult to achieve a proper balance of all the vitamins and minerals in the diet. These situations include:

- episodes of rapid growth, e.g. puberty;
- pregnancy;
- breast-feeding;
- prolonged adherence to a weight-loss programme;
- adherence to a very restricted or fad diet;
- adherence to a vegetarian or vegan diet, unless it is well-balanced;
- old age;
- taking long-term drugs, such as steroids, diuretics (water tablets), anti-epileptic drugs, and possibly the oral contraceptive Pill.

If you fall into any of the above categories, you may need to take a daily multi-vitamin and mineral pill as your nutritional insurance policy! (See Chapter 10.)

8
Controlling your appetite

Certain factors switch the appetite on or off. If it is too readily switched off, we become underweight, and if it is too readily switched on, we become overweight. It is still not yet fully understood how the appetite is controlled. Hunger, caused by lack of food, is the most obvious and indeed most powerful stimulus, but often we have an appetite even though we are not very hungry. In such circumstances, the sight, smell, or indeed taste of food and drink, serve to stimulate our appetite. Something looks delicious, we have eaten it before, and know it tastes delicious, and hey presto, we have an appetite for it.

Social circumstances also dictate our eating habits and appetite. It is customary to offer a drink or a snack to guests and, in some circumstances, it is impolite for them to refuse. Indeed, you have probably broken previous weight-loss diets because of social pressures, such as eating in a restaurant, or eating in a friend's house, where their encouragement, 'go on, it won't hurt', and your response, 'just this once', are the first fatal steps to weight gain. Also, knowledge of what is a good food to eat, and indeed what might be harmful to health, can help to control our appetite.

Certain drugs, including some sex hormones, anti-depressants, and steroids, all serve to stimulate appetite. Emotional factors, in particular recovery from depression, and sometimes response to depressive episodes, may also result in an increased appetite.

CURBING THE APPETITE

So much for what switches it on; what, if anything, switches the appetite off? The sensation obtained from a meal does usually switch the appetite off. This is a combination of factors, including abdominal fullness and an inner feeling of satisfaction, sometimes mingled with the horror of further weight gain. Physical or emotional pain, illness, and some drugs also tell us that now is not the time to eat.

A further important factor is body image. Some people of normal weight feel that they are grossly overweight, and must diet to obtain a 'normal body shape'. Their image is to some degree distorted, and they will all too easily switch their appetite off, rather than let normal hunger and a normal appetite for food develop. At its extreme, this becomes the slimmers' disease, anorexia nervosa. The reverse, thinking you are of normal weight when you are overweight, is, if anything, a rarity. Most of us know when we are overweight.

Unfortunately, there are no magic diets, vitamins, or minerals that will switch your appetite on or off. Slimming drugs do help to suppress the appetite and can be quite successful in assisting short-term weight loss. The tremendous disadvantage is, however, that when the drugs are stopped, the amount of weight regained is almost exactly equal to that lost, and long-term loss from short-term use of appetite-suppressant drugs has yet to be demonstrated.

IT'S A GOOD LIFE

The difference between fat people and thin people is that thin people's bodies tell them when they have had enough to eat. Fat people's bodies just don't know when to say no. For example, it is easy to tell when your body has a fever, is in pain or is tired. These are all experiences we have had that tell us about the body's state at the time, and we do not have difficulty in interpreting them. We have all experienced times of good health, too. If you can't easily remember this, just close your eyes for a moment and recall a time when you felt really well. Probably your weight was less than it is now, and you were physically more active. Perhaps you were on holiday. Just close your eyes and think of that time when you were really well. Remember how your body felt, and perhaps it felt different to how it feels now. The difference is, however, subtle, and not as obvious as being in pain or having a fever.

Eating too much can easily produce abdominal discomfort and a feeling of being stuffed or bloated. This might be associated with physical feelings of lethargy, sleepiness, or a migraine headache, as well as feelings of guilt or depression. Now, if you didn't feel healthy to start with, and if you feel lethargic and bloated most of the time, your body is not going to notice easily when you overeat. What we want to achieve is you losing weight and feeling healthier and having greater awareness of your body. Only in this way will you know when you have overeaten. That feeling of bloating, being stuffed and lethargic, will be so unlike how you normally feel that it will be easy for you to tell when you have eaten too much before you really eat too much. To achieve this, we need to help you to do three things:

● to lose weight
● to eat a diet that is really healthy and nutritious, providing all the vitamins, minerals and protein you need

● to feel really well, having found a diet that suits you.

In this way, if you stray from the healthy diet, you will know immediately; your body will protest and send you a clear message, just as it would if you were too hot or too cold. It is important to learn the skill of knowing when you have had enough!

9
Fibre and weight loss

In recent years, a lot of attention has been given to fibre. A great deal has been said and written, and food manufacturers have been in a hurry to extol the virtues of their food based on its fibre content. However, things are not as simple as they seemed at first. So let's put the record straight and see what part fibre plays in weight loss, health, and appetite control.

WHAT IS FIBRE?

Fibre is the undigestible component of our diet, almost always derived from vegetable produce, and it is those components of the diet that cannot be broken down by the digestive system which in turn pass into the large bowel and contribute to the bulk of faecal waste matter.

WHAT FOODS ARE RICH IN FIBRE?

Fibre is widely distributed in the plant kingdom, and good sources are wholegrains and foods made from them, such as wholemeal bread, coarse oats and sweetcorn. All fruits, and leafy and root vegetables are good sources of fibre. The processing of food, for example turning a whole potato into chips, almost always lowers its fibre content and increases its fat content. That is why consuming refined, processed food makes it easy for you to gain weight.

WHY ARE WE ENCOURAGED TO EAT MORE FIBRE?

People who consume fibre-rich diets do not tend to have many of the diseases associated with the developed countries. Such conditions as coronary artery disease, gallstones, appendicitis, diverticulosis, constipation, and other digestive troubles, as well as varicose veins and obesity, occur less often when large amounts of fibre are consumed in the diet.

ARE THERE DIFFERENT TYPES OF FIBRE?

Yes, fibre is a term for many different substances which have different properties. They all provide bulk in the diet, but some are better at retaining water, and thus softening the stool, which is of benefit for constipation, for example, and others are better at lowering the blood cholesterol level than others. The fibre from fruit and vegetables seems to be particularly beneficial, whereas that from grains may carry fewer benefits.

WHAT HAS FIBRE GOT TO DO WITH WEIGHT LOSS?

Overweight people tend to consume less fibre than their normal-weight counterparts. Concentrating on fibre-rich foods achieves three things. Firstly, fibre-rich foods are more filling and thus satisfying, though of course they take more work to consume as they require more chewing. Secondly, most but not all fibre-rich foods are very nutritious. For example, eating a diet rich in fibre from green vegetables will also provide you with large quantities of vitamins A, B, D and E, magnesium, and a wide range of other minerals. A tablespoonful of bran, which might provide you with the same amount of fibre, is not nearly so nutritious. Thirdly, those of us who are overweight tend to have higher levels of fats in the blood, and fibre-rich foods, when combined with weight loss, can help this enormously and thus lower the risk of heart disease.

ARE THERE ANY SIDE-EFFECTS OF FIBRE?

Surprisingly, yes. Fibre by definition cannot be broken down by our digestive systems, but it can be broken down by the normal healthy bacteria in our large bowel. This may have the side-effect of producing gas and wind. People vary considerably as to how much gas or wind they produce in response to eating different types of foods. Foods that can commonly cause these include onions, cabbage, beans, bran, and large quantities of wholemeal bread. At present, there is no easy way of predicting who may produce gas in response to which foods, and this is a matter for trial and error. This is something you will be exploring in Part Two of the book. This effect, however, tends to minimize as one continues with a high-fibre diet. The body is able to adapt, though this process can take several weeks.

IS IT TRUE THAT BRAN BLOCKS THE ABSORPTION OF CALCIUM?

Yes, bran, wholewheat pasta, chapatis, and large amounts of wholemeal bread contain a substance called phytic acid which blocks the absorption of calcium, magnesium, iron, zinc, copper, and vitamin B_6. It is best not to eat too much of these sorts of fibre in your diet. For this and other reasons we recommend that most of the fibre is obtained from vegetables, salad, and fruit, which does not have this effect, and that you do not simply spoon on dollops of bran in order to increase fibre intake.

Fruit and vegetable fibre is preferable to cereal fibre for the following reasons:

- it generally has fewer calories
- green vegetables have more vitamins and minerals
- it is better at lowering blood cholesterol levels
- higher consumptions of vegetables and fruit are associated with a lower risk of coronary heart disease
- it does not contain phytic acid which blocks the absorption of many important minerals and some vitamins.

Note: In the UK, white bread is fortified with calcium, iron, and some B vitamins. Although it is lower in fibre it may provide more calcium to the body. Thus white bread may be better for those at risk of osteoporosis (thinning of the bones), provided the diet has plenty of fibre and B vitamins from other sources, e.g. green vegetables, salads, and nuts.

10
Becoming a nutritional detective

Getting to know your body is a bit like learning to use a highly complicated machine without a manual. It can be a difficult process and one that requires time and patience.

Although we each have a body, that is where the similarity ends. Each individual body has slightly different requirements. The type of metabolism we have is inherited. There are the lucky ones who have a superbly adapted metabolism: they naturally have a low blood cholesterol level, they can eat almost any type of food, in large quantities, and yet remain healthy and slim. It is highly unlikely that you are reading this book if you happen to be one of the fortunate few!

We have to come to terms with the fact that *most of us have subtle differences which determine the strengths and weaknesses of our make-up*. If you can accept this concept, you will then be able to understand in principle why some people are predisposed to some illnesses or tend to be sensitive to certain types of dietary changes, groups of food, or nutritional defic-iencies. This can also explain why only some people on similar sorts of diet get sick and overweight, while others seem to stay slim and healthy.

ONE BALANCED DIET FOR ALL IS A MYTH

Having accepted the fact that your body is a machine for which you do not have the manual, and that it is not like anyone else's body, what can you do about it? The purpose of the rest of this book is to give you the information you need to compile the missing nutritional manual that will tell you what is just right for your body.

The programme is broken down into three sections. The first part, lasting four weeks, is a 'clean up', which will prepare your body for the second phase, also four weeks. This is a 'trial and error' phase. As you work through the second phase you will be working out the diet that is as near to perfect as you can get it for your own body. During the third phase, lasting two weeks, you will follow a diet that allows you to feel really healthy and to continue losing the unwanted pounds and inches.

GETTING CLUED UP

To become a Nutritional Detective you have to know what you are looking for — the signs and the clues that will eventually lead you to an understanding of your body's individual needs.

It would be a good idea to complete the following questionnaires to give some guide as to your health in a number of important areas.

GENERAL HEALTH AND NUTRITION QUESTIONNAIRE

Let's start with a general questionnaire about your health.

Do you have, or in the last year have you had, any of the following?	YES (score 1 point)	NO (no points)
Anxiety or depression requiring treatment by your doctor		
Prolonged fatigue for no known reason		
High blood pressure		
Recurrent vaginal thrush		
Repeated colds, coughs, sore throats or chest infections		
Premenstrual tension		
Difficulty conceiving		
Repeated mouth ulcers		
Gum disease requiring treatment		
Stomach or duodenal ulcer or severe indigestion requiring treatment by your doctor		
TOTAL SCORE		

This is to see whether any health problems you might have had recently could be affected by your diet, or alcohol and cigarette consumption.

Each one of these common problems could be related to your diet, or alcohol or cigarette consumption. There are of course other reasons for each one, so it is impossible to say exactly how much you can do yourself for any of the conditions mentioned. Certainly if you ticked two or more then it is time to take stock of the situation. Improving the quality of your diet, and reducing your intake of alcohol and cigarettes if you consume them, must help with the problems — and for some it could make a very big difference.

If you have any of the conditions

HEART DISEASE QUESTIONNAIRE

	YES (score 1 point)	NO (no points)
Do you smoke cigarettes or have you *ever* smoked cigarettes?		
Did your mother, father, brother or sister have a heart attack or die from heart disease?		
Are you diabetic requiring insulin, diet, or tablets?		
Have you ever been told by a doctor that your blood pressure was high? (even if you weren't treated)		
If your blood cholesterol has been measured, was it high? (above 5.2mmol/l)		
On average do you drink more than: three units per day (men) two units per day (women) One unit = one glass of wine or half a pint of normal strength beer or one pub measure of spirits or one small sherry or vermouth		
TOTAL SCORE		

listed, your doctor may have already spoken to you about the importance of healthy eating and a healthy lifestyle. If you are receiving medical treatment for any of these conditions, or any other condition for that matter, do check with your doctor before starting this or any other diet. There should not be a problem but it is best to check.

Now let us take a look to see what the future might hold. We have referred before to heart disease and strokes. These remain the biggest killers in most developed countries, and more important the largest preventable cause of premature death (i.e. before the age of 65 years).

This is a questionnaire to assess your risk. Remember that heart disease risk increases substantially if you are seriously overweight or smoke.

If you scored only one point, you probably have only a slightly increased risk of heart disease. If you scored two or more points you should, if you have not already, see your doctor and get further advice from him or her about what you should do to reduce your heart disease and stroke risk. Almost all the risk factors can be easily corrected. No matter what your score, you can still do the diet in Part Two. The only exceptions are diabetics who should obtain advice from their specialist, dietician, or family doctor first.

Finally, lack of exercise is also a risk factor for heart disease but it's relatively small when compared with the others.

Next we are going to look at nutritional deficiencies. Few areas in nutrition and medicine are more hotly debated than whether or not people should take vitamin and mineral supplements. Many experts say no. Many vitamin companies, health food shop owners, and writers on nutrition say yes. As is often the case in this sort of situation, both sides are right to some degree. Certainly, if you are eating a good diet, not smoking cigarettes, consuming little alcohol, are physically and mentally well, aged between 18 and 65 years, and not pregnant or breast-feeding, then you should not need any nutritional supplements. We hope that you fall into this category. If you don't, the answer is a definite 'maybe'! So let us see what the questionnaire can tell us.

Your score will give some idea as to the likelihood of having a deficiency of vitamins or minerals. If there is a deficiency it is important that it is corrected by a good diet and appropriate nutritional supplements. If in doubt, you should of course check this with your family doctor.

In the UK, the commonest deficiencies are of iron and vitamin B. A mild deficiency detected by blood test may not matter if the diet is essentially well-balanced and the person is well. However, if symptoms or signs of deficiency are present, then treatment is indicated.

The signs of iron deficiency are a sore tongue, recurrent mouth ulcers, cracking at the corners of the mouth, flattening of the normal curve of the

HOW TO DETECT YOUR NUTRITIONAL DEFICIENCIES

	YES	NO
Is your complexion very pale?	2	0
If you are a vegetarian or vegan, are you uncertain about how to ensure that your balance of different types of protein is adequate?	1	0
Do you have: • cracking at the corners of the mouth? • cracked or peeling lips? • a sore tongue or repeated mouth ulcers? • very greasy or dry facial skin?	2 2 2 2	0 0 0 0
On average do you smoke more than 10 cigarettes a day?	1	0
Do you drink more than a total of 8 cups of tea and coffee, ordinary or decaffeinated, per day?	1	0
Do you suffer from anxiety or depression requiring treatment by your doctor?	2	0
FOR WOMEN On average, do you drink more than 2 units of alcohol per day?	1	0
Do you suffer from heavy or prolonged periods? (7 days or longer)	1	0
Have you had a baby or been breast-feeding in the last 12 months?	1	0
FOR MEN On average do you drink more than 3 units of alcohol per day?	1	0
TOTAL SCORE		

Score:	*Nutritional deficiencies*
0 – 3	unlikely
4 – 6	possible
7 and over	very likely

Note: The longer any of the above conditions apply, and the less well you feel, the more likely you are to have one or more nutritional deficiencies.

finger or thumb nails, and a pale complexion due to anaemia. If these are present you will need a blood test from your doctor and should not start a special diet without checking with him or her first. A supplement of iron may well be needed and possibly tests to determine the cause of the deficiency.

Lack of vitamin B can produce a variety of symptoms and signs, some of which are similar to iron deficiency. They include redness or greasiness at the side of the nose, cracking at the outer corners of the eyes, or at the corners of the mouth, a sore tongue, recurrent mouth ulcers, and cracking or peeling of the lips. Furthermore, a lack of either iron or vitamin B can cause fatigue, and vitamin B deficiency is sometimes the cause of depression, anxiety, or insomnia.

If you are in doubt about the adequacy of your diet, need to lose more than 10 pounds (4.5kg) in weight, but are otherwise in good health you are probably well advised to take a low-dose multi-vitamin and multi-mineral supplement. If you are generally unwell with any of the above symptoms you should of course consult with your doctor first.

Here is a look at some of the nutritional supplements that are available at either your chemist or health food shop:

Sanatogen; Boots Multi-vitamins; Multi-vitamins BPC
These are cheap multi-vitamin supplements which contain many of the nutrients that might be required by those on a restricted calorie intake.

Sanatogen With Iron; Boots Multi-vitamins With Iron
Multi-vitamins with iron are a good idea if you have heavy periods, particularly if you are a vegetarian.

Health Insurance Plus; Cantamega 2000; Quest-One-A-Day
These and other similar products are all strong multi-vitamin multi-mineral supplements. They are quite expensive and contain substantially more than is usually needed. It may be a good idea to take them if you are ill or if you are a heavy alcohol consumer but they should not be routinely necessary.

Optivite
This is a strong multi-vitamin, multi-mineral supplement of proven efficacy in the treatment of pre-menstrual tension. It is also rather costly and too strong for routine use by those on weight-loss programmes.

Evening Primrose Oil (e.g. Efamol) is also helpful for PMT but does not contain any vitamins or minerals. It is a specialized oil supplement.

Diet Balance

This is a new multi-vitamin, multi-mineral supplement which contains a wide range of vitamins and minerals at levels very close to those provided by a healthy diet. It is moderately priced. It is designed to be taken by people who are on a weight-loss diet, in order that they get the correct daily balance of vitamins and minerals.

It is important to remember that there is no special supplement of vitamins, minerals, or anything else for that matter, that will melt your excess weight away. There is no substitute for a well-balanced calorie-reduced diet. It is important that those who are on such diets long term take care to ensure an adequate intake of essential nutrients.

11
Food allergies and how to detect them

After the question of nutritional deficiencies, few subjects are more topical than food allergy and intolerance. For many years, the majority of doctors questioned whether food allergies occurred at all, but things have changed, particularly in the last decade. Many of us are aware that some foods agree with us and some do not. This is part of the individual nature of our body's metabolism.

Part of our individuality is determined by the functioning of the immune system. This system produces white cells and antibodies that help us resist infection. It has a particular quality to recognize substances as being either 'self', i.e. part of the normal body's metabolism, or 'non-self', i.e. a foreign substance from outside. Some individuals may become unusually sensitive to such foreign non-self substances, and this in turn can cause an allergic reaction. Good examples are grass-pollen producing hay fever, some constituents of perfume or make-up producing contact dermatitis, and sensitivity to gluten — a

protein found in wheat — producing coeliac disease. In this latter condition, gluten (which is also found in oats, barley, and rye) produces damage to the lining of the bowel, preventing normal absorption of nutrients from the diet. These are all classical examples of an allergy.

Sometimes, changes in the blood, either in the white cells or in the blood proteins, i.e. antibodies, cannot be detected in people who react adversely to foods. In such cases, the term 'food intolerance' is then used. It is becoming increasingly appreciated that while food allergies may be relatively rare, food intolerance may be much more common, and usually produces milder symptoms.

Conditions in which food allergies are known to play a part include eczema, asthma, nettle-rash (urticaria), rhinitis, swelling of the lips or throat, rheumatoid arthritis, and migraine.

Food intolerance may certainly aggravate a common bowel disorder called irritable bowel syndrome. In this condition, the sufferer experiences either constipation or diarrhoea, often in association with excessive abdominal bloating and sometimes pains, usually cramp-like and situated either in the middle or lower part of the abdomen. This is a common disorder, affecting some 11 per cent of the population. Such symptoms may be present for a few days or weeks and then clear up but in many, the symptoms are persistent.

There is no satifactory drug treatment for irritable bowel syndrome, and a variety of diets have been recommended. At one time it was thought that high-fibre diets containing bran would be successful, but this has not proved to be the case. More recent research has suggested that approximately two-thirds of individuals may improve by changing their diet and avoiding certain foods. Constituents of the diet such as milk, bread, cheese, butter, tea, coffee, alcohol, and even cigarettes have the potential to aggravate or cause the symptoms of irritable bowel syndrome.

A leading group of doctors who have researched this condition are at Addenbrooke's Hospital in Cambridge. Their research, led by Dr John Hunter, Consultant Gastroenterologist, revealed the connection between diet and irritable bowel syndrome (IBS). Surprisingly, one of the commonest foods found to cause IBS was wheat, especially in the form of bran and wholemeal bread. This was a real turn up for the books, and is an observation still not accepted by all medical practitioners. Of course, not everybody with irritable bowel syndrome has food intolerances, nor are they going to be intolerant of every food they eat. Sometimes it is just one food, or perhaps three or four, and this is yet another example of individuality.

Migraine headaches are another condition that need a mention. A severe headache with nausea or vomiting, and often with disturbance of vision or sensitivity to light, typify a migraine. It is now widely accepted that such headaches can be precipitated by foods as well as stress, the oral contraceptive Pill, and the build-up to a period. The commonest foods to cause a migraine are alcoholic drinks, cheese, pickled foods, chocolate, tea, coffee, and foods rich in yeast such as Marmite and savoury foods or sauces containing yeast extract (look at the label).

The great unanswered question about food allergy and intolerance is what causes it? Many children develop allergies in the first few weeks or months of life, and often these improve as the years go by. Many cases of childhood eczema may be due to allergy to cow's milk, but some 50 per cent or so may clear up quite spontaneously, without any change in diet. This is just the newly-born body becoming acclimatized to the type of diet and foodstuffs that we now eat. Food allergy and intolerance have certainly become much more common in the adult population, and the reason is unknown. Perhaps changes in the type of foods we eat, exposure to environmental chemicals and pollutants, and changes in the type of infections we now experience have caused this.

Each of the eight conditions listed in the questionnaire can be caused by factors other than food allergy or intolerance. So if you marked just one, food allergy or intolerance is a possibility but not certain. If you marked two, the chances are definitely increasing, and with three or more it is well worth considering a change of diet to see if this helps.

ALLERGY QUESTIONNAIRE

	YES (score 1 point)	NO (no score)
Do you suffer from:		
migraine		
asthma		
rhinitis/chronic catarrh/blocked, stuffy or running nose		
eczema not due to a contact allergy (such as detergents or perfume)		
nettle-rash (urticaria), or hives		
angioedema (sudden swelling of the lip, face or throat after eating certain foods)		
rheumatoid arthritis		
irritable bowel syndrome or spastic colon; constipation, diarrhoea or a mixture of the two		
Have you suffered from any of these badly in the past?		
Do/did your parents suffer from asthma, eczema, nettle-rash, or hay fever?		
TOTAL SCORE		

This is one of the key points about the diet in Part Two. The foods that commonly cause or aggravate these conditions are for the most part excluded from the diet. Previous weight-loss or crash diets may well have failed in the short or long term because they did not take into account problems you might have had with food allergy or intolerance. Do not think that you have to have one of these conditions in order to do the diet — you don't. You should be starting to realize that there are many ways in which improving your diet can help.

Also in Part Two you will learn much more about some of the suspect foods including sugar, animal fats, dairy products, wheat and other grains, tea, coffee, chocolate, yeast products, and alcohol — as well as cigarettes.

12
Diets in practice

The diet that we eat is influenced by a variety of different factors, both consciously and subconsciously. No single factor is dominant and all are important to varying degrees, depending upon the individual, and the circumstances in which she or he lives.

It would be nice to think that if people knew the correct diet for them, particularly the correct diet for weight loss, they would simply go and follow it, and that would be the end of obesity. Little could be further from the truth. Many of us have tried to lose weight and failed miserably for one reason or another. Success is usually followed by failure until the next successful dietary regime is found. We can only break out of this vicious circle by understanding the factors that influence the dietary choices we make.

THE KEY FACTORS

Cost

Most if not all of us run our lives on some kind of budget. We have money for clothes, the housekeeping, for paying the mortgage or rent, the house bills, car, and holidays. Instinctively we know which foods are expensive, and which are cheap, and purchase foods using this knowledge. In the UK the current average expenditure on food is just under £2 per person per day. In addition, for every £1 we spend on food, we spend a further 50p on alcohol and 22p on cigarettes.

On the weight-loss programme in Part Two, you should not spend any more than usual on your week's shopping. You may find that you spend a little more on food, but savings are made because of the reduction in expenditure on alcohol and perhaps cigarettes.

Tradition

We are, by and large, creatures of habit. When looked at on a year-to-year basis, our diets may vary little. There are of course substantial variations in dietary habits from country to country, and from family to family. Dietary habits are also influenced to some degree by social class; for example, those from a working class background tend to eat less fruit and vegetables than others.

To some degree we tend to eat the foods that we ate as children. Only in more recent years have our dietary habits changed. From 1976 to 1984, all social groups made small but significant reductions in the consumption of refined sugar, saturated animal fats, and white breads.

We have on average increased our consumption of fruit and vegetables by approximately 10 per cent, with the exception of those in the unemployed and working class categories. Unfortunately, people in this latter group have *decreased* their consumption by 10 per cent, thus widening an important dietary difference between the social groups. Having a good consumption of fruit and vegetables is a very important part of a healthy weight-loss programme.

To lose weight means changing your diet, and to do that means changing some of your shopping habits. Buying this week what you bought last week is only going to end in failure. The changes are coming.

Choice and availability

In times of hardship, as in the depression in the 1920s and 30s and rationing during the 1940s and 50s, there has not always been a great choice of food. Nowadays, in developed countries, we live in times of plenty, and every supermarket and greengrocer is offering an ever-increasing choice of food products. It has never been easier to change and choose a healthier weight-loss programme. Lack of choice is rarely a limiting factor. We have taken great care to make sure that the foods recommended on the diet are all widely available, little influenced by seasonal variations.

Taste

Of course, the taste of a food is an overriding factor. Nowadays, in times of plenty, we naturally eat only foods that we enjoy the taste of. With so much choice we almost never have to eat foods that we don't enjoy.

Tolerance

As well as you liking the food, the food has to like you. This is a whole subject in itself, which we have already mentioned. There are many foods that are commonly not well tolerated, and the basic structure of the diet is not only to remove the calorie-rich foods that cause obesity, but also those foods that are commonly not tolerated. In the long run, you are best to avoid or severely limit those foods to which you are intolerant. The careful design of the diet will allow you to determine for yourself which foods you can tolerate, and which you cannot.

Convenience

We do not just mean convenience

foods, but the convenience of eating a meal in relation to the time allowed, and the situation. Our expectations of achievement have been steadily rising. We have become busier and more efficient and productive with each passing decade, and this has meant cutting down on the time spent on more mundane activities. We no longer grow, harvest and prepare all our own food. It is more convenient to have it grown for us, harvested for us, and in some cases, meals actually prepared for us.

If your life is so rushed that you only have five to ten minutes for lunch, and your body knows that you have to consume at least 300–400 calories in order to make it through until the evening, it is going to look for a very convenient solution, and that means, high-calorie, low-volume food that is readily available, such as a chunky cheese sandwich, or worse still, a chocolate bar. None of these foods are going to help you to lose weight, though they are all quick and convenient. To achieve lasting weight loss, you are going to need to set aside time for the preparation and consumption of food, and that may mean altering your lifestyle.

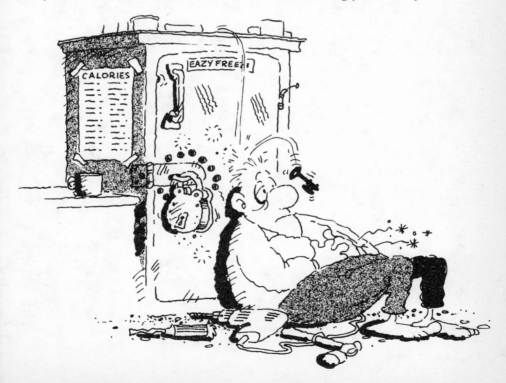

Knowledge

Last, but by no means least, comes knowledge of what is a healthy diet. For hundreds and indeed thousands of years, this knowledge has only been intuitive, passed on from generation to generation. Different cultures have had different views of what a healthy diet is. With the arrival of scientific methods in the twentieth century, we have been able to determine the essential nature of a healthy diet, and with it make dietary changes based on knowledge.

This book will provide you not only with a healthy weight-loss programme that will suit your metabolism, but also the knowledge that is necessary to help you adhere to it.

The knowledge is not just dry pages of fact after fact, but knowledge gained from analysing your first-hand experience. You are going to find out what foods suit you, and turn that knowledge into a long-lasting, successful weight-loss programme.

Just as we are all different in our body weight and metabolism, so the type of diet we eat is influenced by factors which differ from person to person. For some, cost may not be a factor, but for many it is. For others, convenience and speed of preparation is everything in their hurried lifestyles. For those of us with children, we may have more reason than just our own good health to consider in trying to find out what a healthy diet is.

13
Mental well-being

Most of us have dieted at some time in our lives, and have been able to stick to the new regime quite rigidly for a little while. It is not your ability to diet that is in question. However, it is a staggering fact that 9 out of 10 people who successfully lose weight on a 'diet' put the weight back on again afterwards. It is important to identify why this occurs, and then to find a solution for each reason. This will mean that you can confidently go ahead and lose weight, knowing that you are able to maintain the weight loss afterwards.

The way we are feeling mentally may have a direct effect on our shape. If you are one of the comfort eaters and find that your mood patterns have a direct effect on your eating habits then it must be a good idea for you to examine just how the various moods you experience affect your eating habits.

See how you get on with the following questions: if you answer 'yes' to one or more, then we have some further work to do in this area! In theory, a positive answer to one or more of the following situations

could open the door to you regaining weight after this diet. All the questions represent potential weaknesses in our ability to stick to diets. Those questions that you answered positively may well prove to be a threat to your ability to maintain a good figure and an optimum state of health.

In an attempt to prevent you regaining the unwanted pounds we have looked at each individual question and made some suggested solutions.

DIET HISTORY QUESTIONNAIRE

Question
Can you manage to stick to a weight-loss diet when you have a defined time period, i.e. the three weeks until your holiday, or if you have to fit into certain clothes for a special occasion which is soon to be upon you, and do you generally find it difficult to stick to a diet for a longer period?

Reasoning
If you are going on to a diet which involves being very restricted for

choice, and in some cases, missing out meals altogether, you are perfectly normal if you find it difficult to stick to this in the long term. It may be all very well when you have a goal in sight and you have only a few weeks to get through. However, in order to be successful in the long term, you need to learn how to change your eating habits permanently, to suit your own body. You need to be on a diet that is healthy, well-balanced, and that you enjoy and makes you feel good.

Question

Does your eating pattern change according to how you are faring emotionally? For example, if your love life is thriving you can manage to maintain your diet, but as soon as there is an upset, or things are not going so smoothly, then your dietary resolutions go out of the window?

Reasoning

If you fit into this category, you are more than likely a comfort eater. It would seem that you have some undesirable dietary habits lurking in the wings. At the first sign of the emotional see-saw that life so often presents, you go scurrying off for the goodies that give you comfort.

By changing your dietary habits and helping to keep your blood sugar on a more constant level, we would hope to have you in better physical and mental shape. As a result you should feel good enough to communicate your way through whatever problem presents itself, and bring about a fast resolution. If you don't feel so good,

the problems tend to look larger. Once you feel 'on top' physically and mentally, you will find that the problems seem far more manageable.

Question

Do you find that you tend to generally eat more, or crave sweet food more, when you are feeling tired or have gone without food for a long time?

Reasoning

At times when you have been very busy and may have missed or delayed a meal, your blood glucose levels can fall. The brain needs glucose to function and the body reacts causing you to feel faint, sweaty and light-headed, and to experience difficulty in concentrating. This produces a desire to eat sweet snack–foods. Apart from changing your diet, it would be a great idea if you could grant yourself a little more importance, and make sure you avoid getting overtired or missing meals, when at all possible.

Question

When the heat is on at work and you are required to work longer hours, are you unable to maintain your eating pattern?

Reasoning

It is obviously more difficult to set aside time for meal planning if you happen to be going through a heavy time at work. However, if you know exactly what you need to be eating it is far easier to ensure that your body gets what it needs. In the menu section, you will find a series of suggestions for packed lunches, and also for acceptable meals that you should be able to buy from snack bars or small supermarkets in the vicinity of your workplace.

Question

Do you often feel stressed and over-stretched in life, and during these times find that you tend to eat more, particularly the foods of the fattening variety?

Reasoning

Taking on a bit more than you can happily cope with in life can result in feelings of distress and overwhelm you to some degree. When your attention is so wrapped around the problems or situations in hand it is easy to lose sight of your own body's requirements. Taking the example of the working mother: she usually has so many roles to fulfil that her needs very definitely take a back seat.

If you are in this position it is important to take stock of what you have taken on. You have to realize that to a large degree you are the master of your own destiny. Your mental and physical well-being are vital, as without them you will not be able to fulfil the tasks you have before you. You must make sure that you only take upon yourself those things that you know you can manage comfortably. You have to learn to say 'no'. It is very important for the sake of your own sanity. It would be a very good investment for you to set aside time for yourself each day, even if it's just time for a bit of personal planning and some gentle exercise.

Question

Do you just drift along and accept what comes your way, rather than having specific goals that you are working towards in life?

Reasoning

Having a direction in life is very important. If you don't already have goals that you are aiming for (at work, at home, and in leisure), it is advisable for you to spend some time and work out what you really want to achieve. Then work out a way that you can attain that goal over a period of time. If you have trouble sorting out what your exact goals are, try thinking back to some time in your childhood when you had dreams and aspirations. You can usually find some of your basic goals became apparent during this period of time. There is nothing so soul-destroying as living from day to day with no purpose. It's hardly surprising that you would turn to food for comfort under these circumstances.

Question

Are you aware that you eat differently at certain times of the month and perhaps even crave sweet food before your period arrives?

Reasoning

If you are not aware that your eating habits change depending on the time of your menstrual cycle, it would be worth keeping a diary for a few months to check. It is very common for eating habits to change during the week or two leading up to your period, particularly cravings for sweet foods.

The hormone changes that occur are closely linked to nutritional changes in the body. Blood sugar levels and nutritional requirements do fluctuate, and so it is particularly important to be aware of what is occurring and to be educated to the point where you know how to treat your body at any given time of the month.

Question

Do you sometimes find that you are doing very little in the way of physical exercise for several weeks at a time?

Reasoning

Exercise is an extremely important tool in increasing your body's metabolic rate. There are few ways of increasing the speed at which your body metabolizes food, but this is a very valuable one. If your exercise programme has lapsed it is time you reinstated it on a regular basis. If you do not participate in regular exercise, then you should begin some sort of exercise programme at the same time as you begin your diet. You would be advised to read Chapter 15 before choosing the type of exercise that would be best for you.

Question

When you are busy and time is at a premium, do you end up 'snacking' rather than bothering to have proper meals?

Reasoning

It's all too easy to get carried away with the business of everyday life, and to put your own requirements to the bottom of the pile. You must appreciate that the health and well-being of your mind and body are of paramount importance. If you regularly take snacks instead of eating properly, you will deny yourself the important nutrients that your body requires. Ultimately you will not feel so well, and will find it difficult to maintain your figure as a result.

Question

Do you sometimes eat through boredom?

Reasoning

There is really no need to be bored these days as there is so much going on. You must make sure that you are occupied to the point where you do not feel bored. Many pounds of weight are put on through 'private' eating sessions. Don't sit alone. Either visit friends, or invite them to your place. Join evening classes or some sort of club that could further one of your dormant hobbies.

Question

Is your home environment fairly disorderly?

Reasoning

If the answer to this is 'yes', you will be surprised how much better you will feel once you have carried out a clearing-up project. It's like mental spring-cleaning! You should use the time to have a good clear out, and then implement new systems, e.g.

new homes for different sorts of clothes and belongings, and perhaps a formal filing system, if you do not already have one, for your loose papers. There is nothing like putting off the chores to send you diving into the biscuit box or cookie jar!

Question

Can you think of many projects, either at work or at home, that you have begun, but not completed?

Reasoning

If you fall into this category you should make a list of all the outstanding and unfinished projects you have on the go. Begin the list with the projects that have been waiting to be finished for the longest period of time. Decide on a time each week to work on finishing off projects, and make a start at the beginning of the list, and work your way through it, ticking off the completed projects as you finish them. Pay particular attention not to take on any new tasks during this period. Simply concentrate on getting through your list. You will find that you feel much better once you get started, and that need to snack and pick at extra food between meals will disappear.

Question

When you are feeling worried or anxious do you noticeably eat more as a comfort?

Reasoning

It's fairly natural to either stop eating well at times when you feel nervous or anxious, or to go to the other extreme and over-indulge. If you do find that you over-indulge you must make a concerted effort to curb this.

Very often you can't change the situation immediately. You can talk about it to a close friend, though, which very often helps to alleviate some tension. You could work out how you could help to ease the situation and subsequently make yourself feel better. Whether it's a long-term or short-term problem, you will find that gentle exercise and relaxation through yoga will be beneficial to you mentally and physically, and we always find that a good massage goes a long way to easing tension and making you feel better.

RELAXATION

Taking time out just to relax each day is highly desirable, even if you have a really comfortable place to lie down take fifteen to twenty minutes. Find a really comfortable place to lay down and cut loose. Day-dreaming is very therapeutic. Just let your mind wander to sunnier climates and pretend you are indulging in your favourite pursuit, or as an alternative you can concentrate on getting each part of your body to relax. Begin with your toes on the left foot, then the toes on the right foot, followed by each foot separately, and then slowly work your way up to your face and head. There is an art in doing this, and it does take a bit of practice. You should relax for a while when you have finished before rushing off to get on with life. Once you are practised at this sort of relaxation you will feel quite refreshed afterwards. Your mental attitude and well-being has great influence over how much you indulge, so relaxation should become an important feature in your day, to help you feel good.

14
Controlling sugar cravings

All the new year's resolutions in the world will not necessarily curb your cravings for sweet food. As firmly as you may resolve to leave the sweet foods alone, when the 'munchies' arrive, your resistance is often overwhelmed without too much difficulty. There are good reasons for this mechanism. You can rest assured that you do not give in just because you have a weak constitution!

A craving for sweet foods can be the body's way of saying that the blood glucose level is low. While a sugary snack may temporarily raise blood sugar levels, it is certainly not the long-term answer as the refined foods soon metabolize and the blood sugar levels will fall rapidly. Nothing short of changed dietary habits and a good vitamin and mineral balance will resolve the problem in the long term.

SUGAR CRAVING — THE PROBLEM

As a result of treating thousands of patients with sugar cravings, and discovering that nearly 80 per cent of a group of 1,000 women with premenstrual syndrome also claimed to be suffering with sugar cravings, WNAS undertook a national study to determine the degree of the problem in general. From the 500 women who were questioned all over England and Scotland the following facts emerged:

- 72 per cent of the women said they would like to consume less sugar
- 60 per cent admitted that consuming sugar was a problem
- just under 40 per cent admitted that weight gain was the worst problem created by their sugar cravings
- 23 per cent said they became noticeably moody and irritable shortly after consuming sugar
- 78 per cent most of all wanted to eat chocolate.

SUGAR'S SWEET SECRETS QUESTIONNAIRE

The following questions relate to your consumption of sugar-containing foods over the last seven days. Before answering them, just

Over the last seven days:	LOW (none/1)	MED. (2 or 3)	HIGH (4 or more)
How many chocolate bars or portions/servings of chocolate or sweets have you eaten?	1	2	3
How many portions of cakes, desserts or puddings, or 'portions' of biscuits (1 biscuit counts as ¼ portion) have you eaten?	1	2	3
How many cans or bottles of non-low-calorie soft drinks or servings of ice-cream have you eaten?	1	2	3
How many portions have you eaten, either shop-bought or home-made, of foods containing sugar, e.g. fruit pies, desserts, custard?	1	2	3
How many cups of tea, coffee, chocolate or other drinks *with sugar* did you consume per day?	1	2	3
TOTAL			

spend a minute thinking back over the last week.

Now answer the questions. Ring the grade that applies to you, then total up your score.

    5   Low consumer
6 – 10   Moderate consumer
11 – 15   High consumer

DIETARY FACTORS

An inadequate diet, as well as large amounts of sugar, can also lead to craving, which then results in some very unpleasant symptoms:

- nervousness and anxiety
- palpitations
- headaches

- dizziness and fainting
- weight gain.

It is important not to skip meals as this will serve to make matters worse. If you miss breakfast, energy levels tend to crash by mid-morning, with symptoms including craving for sweet foods.

When sugar cravings are severe, it is better to eat smaller meals more often, as this also helps to balance blood sugar levels.

Large amounts of coffee, alcohol and cigarettes as well as sugar serve only to aggravate the problem, particularly if they are taken in place of a meal.

THE 'MAGIC' MINERAL

Chromium is a mineral which is thought to play a very important part in the regulation of blood sugar in the body. Only minute quantities are required by us and a lifetime supply of chromium weighs only a fraction of one ounce. Although small, this tiny

MICHELE FLETCHER

Michele had been two stones (28lb/12.5kg) overweight since her late teens.

'I have had a weight problem for 15 years. I was 2 stones overweight. I lost weight after the birth of my first child and then I put the weight back on again. With me, diets went out of the window because I had pre-menstrual tension and severe sweet cravings. This lasted for 3 weeks per month and so I was only able to diet properly for 1 week out of every 4.

'It didn't seem worth dieting for only 1 week. I found this very depressing.

'I tried Weight Watchers and other low-calorie diets. Many of them were successful for a short while but the weight soon went on again. I found losing weight progressively difficult after having the children.

'I went on the WNAS programme. The first two weeks were a bit rough. I had cut out all grains and foods containing yeast, plus sweet foods. I was amazed that I managed to stick to the diet and keep off sweet foods. I took the supplement Sugar Factor which I am sure curbed my cravings for sweet foods. I haven't binged since I began the WNAS diet and the Sugar Factor.

'The thrush and cystitis I was experiencing chronically before the diet have cleared up. My migraines are much better now also and my PMT has gone. All this *and I managed to lose 2 stones which has stayed off*. I do half an hour's exercise per day now and I feel much better for it.'

amount of chromium has a critical part to play. Babies are born with a good supply of chromium, but the level tends to fall as we get older.

It is difficult to test reliably for chromium deficiency, as most laboratories are not equipped to perform accurate tests. However, in view of the low toxicity of chromium, when suffering with sugar cravings it may be worth trying chromium supplements as a way of overcoming the sweet cravings.

Chromium supplements have been shown to help stop the swings both high and low in blood glucose levels. A well-balanced diet, rich in complex carbohydrates such as vegetables, fruits, beans, nuts and seeds, as well as protein-rich foods, also helps

---

SUZANNE CHAPMAN

Suzanne began having problems with her weight after her pregnancy just over two years ago. She went from a size 8 to nearly a size 16 and was unable to lose any of the excess weight.

'I was pretty desperate to lose weight. I cut out all fizzy drinks and chocolate for 5 months but I did not manage to lose any weight. I felt hungry, miserable and frustrated. I used to get through 7–8 big bottles of Cream Soda per week and at least 3 chocolate bars per day, as well as sweets and sugar in tea.

'Looking back I now realize my diet affected my moods. I used to hit out at my husband and throw things at him. I felt so upset with myself that I used to go out for a drive to cool off.

'I found the WNAS programme took some getting used to for the first few weeks. Once I got used to the diet it was plain sailing. I lost 2 stones in weight over a four month period and the weight loss has been maintained.

'I took the supplement Sugar Factor which curbed my sugar cravings very quickly. I feel much healthier now both physically and mentally. I'm right back to a size 10.

'The main thing that kept me going was that I kept reading about people who had been successful on the WNAS programme and seeing them on TV.

'I found I could not tolerate sweet foods or foods containing wholewheat or yeast very well and soon after I eliminated these from my diet I felt much better. Apart from the weight loss I feel much more relaxed. I swim a lot and walk much more. In general I feel happier with myself at eight and a half stone and I feel I am able to get more out of life.'

enormously.

The Women's Nutritional Advisory Service have formulated a special supplement especially to help deal with the problem of sugar cravings, called Sugar Factor. This supplement is designed as a temporary nutritional prop while you are making dietary adjustments. It is available by mail order, details of which are on page 234.

15
Paying attention to the bodywork

If your aim is to look good and feel good, then you need to follow some sort of exercise programme. The positive value of exercise should not be under-estimated. It is a fact that exercise is of general benefit to people of all ages because it is necessary for the optimum function, structure and preservation of muscles, bones, joints, and the heart. Regular exercise can improve the quality of and extend an active life, and plays a vital part in the prevention of many chronic conditions.

Weight loss has been found to have a direct relationship to the amount of exercise taken. The increased energy expenditure of exercise assists in weight reduction. Obesity is associated with a raised blood cholesterol, heart disease, and high blood pressure. Exercise lowers the risk or effect of these conditions aside from any effect of diet or weight loss. Vigorous exercise reduces the risk of an overweight person contracting one of these conditions to almost the same level as a non-overweight person.

HOW DOES EXERCISE HELP PROMOTE WEIGHT LOSS?

The energy you use in the process of exercising burns up extra calories and may help to increase your resting metabolic rate. Providing you stick to your diet, and don't consume lots of extra calories, you get into what is called calorie deficit. This means that if you do an hour's vigorous exercise instead of sitting in a chair for an hour, you could burn up an extra 100–200 calories which would not have otherwise been used up. As long as you also stick to your diet, weight loss will occur.

WHAT SORT OF EXERCISE?

Physical activity is an important factor in maintaining fitness and energy balance. You should begin exercising at the correct pace. If the exercise programme you choose is too vigorous for you it will only leave you feeling tired, achy and disappointed. If, on the other hand, your exercises are insufficient to stimulate your limb and heart muscles, thus providing aerobic exercise, then you will be effectively wasting your time.

What is aerobic exercise?

Contrary to popular belief, aerobic exercise does not necessarily mean jumping around in your local keep fit class for an hour. Aerobic exercise is exercise that stimulates the large groups of muscles in your body, getting them to contract rhythmically. Over a period of time these muscles, including the heart which is a muscular organ, become more efficient. Eventually the heart in particular can work more slowly, but with increased efficiency. Once in this condition, you will usually experience an increased sense of well-being, on both a physical and a mental level. It also means that your chances of having heart disease are less.

In order to reap the benefits that aerobic exercise can provide, you have to exercise regularly, and for at least half an hour each time. You need to engage in aerobic exercise three to four times per week in order to make physical progress. Apart from those exercise classes that are called 'Aerobics', there are many other forms of exercise that qualify. For example, brisk walking, swimming, cycling, and jogging are all aerobic exercises.

Where do you start?

In order for us to assess where you should make a start you need to answer the questionnaire overleaf, unless you are already on a really good exercise programme, which gives you at least three half-hour sessions of vigorous exercise per week.

HOW TO CHOOSE YOUR EXERCISE PLAN

More than 30 per cent overweight and unfit

If you are more than 30 per cent overweight and you get puffed out easily, do little or no exercise, and consider yourself unfit, you should begin by following the recommendations gradually. Begin by exercising moderately for 5–10 minutes per day, and build up gradually over a period of a month. Walking and swimming are good stamina–building exercises.

10–30 per cent overweight and not as fit as you should be

If you are between 10 and 30 per cent overweight, and similarly you get puffed easily, do little or no exercise, and consider yourself unfit, you too should begin by exercising gently. If you are less than 20 per cent overweight, you will be able to increase your pace that much faster. You should begin by going for a walk each day for half an hour or so. Gradually, you will need to increase your pace to the point where you are walking briskly and you can feel your heart pumping away efficiently, but not to the point where you feel at all overwhelmed. You should still be able to talk whilst you are exercising; that is a good guide to know whether you are overdoing it or not.

Up to 10 per cent overweight and exercise occasionally

If you are a little overweight for your height and are doing some moderate exercise each week, but agree that it's not really optimum and you could be doing a lot better, you need to follow an 'improver' programme. This will involve stepping up your pace gradually, and increasing the number of times you exercise per week. Swimming is great training exercise. It is a good way to get all your muscles working without experiencing the aches afterwards.

EXERCISE QUESTIONNAIRE

(Tick any answer that applies to you now)	TICK
Are you more than 30 per cent or more over your ideal weight? (see page 30 for weight chart)	
Are you more than 20 per cent over your ideal weight?	
Are you more than 10 per cent over your ideal weight?	
Do you currently do no exercise whatsoever?	
Do you currently do some gentle exercise occasionally?	
Do you exercise once or twice per week in a formal setting?	
Do you exercise more than three times per week for more than half an hour each time?	
Do you get puffed out easily?	
Can you run up and down the stairs without panting?	
Which would you describe yourself as: • very unfit • unfit • not as fit as you should be • moderately fit • fit • in excellent physical condition!	

Overweight but fit

If you are overweight, but are happy with the exercises you do at least three times per week, then far be it from us to interfere — continue, you are obviously doing a good job!

ENJOY YOUR EXERCISE TIME

It is really important that you look upon your exercise time as an enjoyable experience. If you do not select the sort of exercise that you enjoy, there isn't very much hope of you sticking to it, is there? Some of us are sporty and others just are not. There is no point arranging to play squash if you really dislike the game, or vowing to go for a jog each day, if you hate running. So do select the sort of exercise that you like.

Also, you can vary the type of exercise you do during the week. For example, you may like to swim on Mondays and Fridays, play squash on Wednesdays, and go for a long brisk walk or jog on Saturdays and Sundays. There is no reason why you can't do the same exercises each day, but obviously increasing the amount gently. The only reason we suggest you vary it a bit is to prevent boredom. Here's to a new you!

PART TWO

16
Preparing for the diet

This is not a diet to launch into as soon as you have finished reading about it. This time, a little less haste and a little more care and planning is necessary.

First of all, you have to finish reading up to page 100, and don't skip any pages, and don't read any further either, because thereafter you read one page per day.

WHO SHOULD NOT DO THE DIET

There are certain people who should not attempt this diet. For some individuals, a substantial weight loss or sudden change in diet is inadvisable.

You should thus not attempt the diet:

- if you are underweight
- if you are already on a diet from your doctor or a dietitian
- if you have any serious illness
- if you are pregnant or breast-feeding
- if you have diabetes — unless your doctor approves.

PREPARATION STEPS

- You are going to need to buy some bathroom scales if you haven't got any, or if the ones you have got aren't accurate, because each day you are going to weigh yourself to the nearest pound (0.5kg). The best time to do this is first thing in the morning, after going to the bathroom, wearing your night-clothes or nothing at all, but keep it the same every day. Of course, you can take your clothes off and wash them, or change them as appropriate!

- You are going to need a pair of kitchen scales or letter scales to weigh your food accurately. We are sorry to be negative but, quite simply, we just don't trust you, or rather we don't think that you yet trust yourself to know exactly what 4oz (115g) of lean meat, 6oz (170g) of fish, 2oz (55g) of carrots, or 4oz (115g) peas really look like. By the end of the diet you will know exactly what they look like, and you won't need to weigh them.

This is part of the knowledge that you are going to have, and it is a very important part. Classically, overweight people under-estimate the volume of food and the amount of calories that they consume. We need to break that dangerous little habit and the only way is by education. A pair of kitchen scales will do that easily. Make sure the scales read accurately and by at least half-ounce or 10-gram divisions.

- You will need some organization. The best time to do this diet is when you have two months un-complicated by going on holiday, moving house, changing your job, doing large amounts of business travel, or entertaining at home or at work. If you want to change your weight, you are going to have to change your diet, and to do that you are going to need a regular, orderly lifestyle. If you have a rapidly changing lifestyle, it is going to be very difficult indeed to make changes in your diet as well. You need to be in control of, and not controlled by, the day's events.

- An absolutely essential ingredient is time. You are going to need time to go shopping twice a week, time to prepare your food, time to eat it, and five to ten minutes at the beginning of each day to read a page of the book, record your weight, and record any symptoms you're experiencing. At the end of each week, which we suggest is a Saturday, you will need a little extra time to review your progress, and work out your weight loss for that week.

PREPARATION CHECKLIST

Tick when done:
- Bathroom scales, working, or new ones purchased: ....
- Kitchen scales, working, or new ones purchased: ....
- Daily schedule organized so that lifestyle is regular and orderly. Go over any problem areas with your partner. ....
- Time set aside for preparation and consumption of breakfast, lunch and supper: ....
- Go through the kitchen examining all the food in the larder, refrigerator and freezer. If it is on the forbidden list, either throw it out, give it to the children/cat/dog, or, in the case of frozen food, put it at the back of the freezer out of reach. It is a good idea to clear a shelf in the fridge for *your* particular foods, though many of the foods that you will be eating can be easily incorporated into your family's diet. When you have done all this, mark it as done. ....

- You will also need some willpower, but we are not asking for very much. We are sure you have tried to lose weight before, and have had some success and some failures. There were good reasons for the failures, we are sure. We can't control all of these, but the one that we can control is your knowledge of what a healthy weight-loss programme is, and what foods suit your body's metabolism. Armed with this information, we are sure that you have the willpower to succeed.

Finally, tell your family and friends that you are starting a diet. Maybe they will want to join in too. Doing the diet with someone else or in a small group will help you to be successful. But take care; not everybody's response to certain parts of the diet will be the same. That's the whole secret. This diet will determine what's right for you, and only you can find that out.

17
Vital dieting tips

In the fight against obesity you have, no doubt, often regarded yourself as your own worst enemy. Equally, you can be your own best friend. But to do so, you are going to have to treat yourself, your eating habits, and the question of weight loss quite seriously. This is not a matter of just sticking doggedly to a particular diet, but also of looking at your eating habits. Your day-by-day programme will take you through the necessary steps but, first, here are some important tips on the subject of food.

- **Start the diet when you are ready to do so.** You are going to need time. This is not a diet to do in a hurry, and it is certainly not a crash diet.

- **Plan ahead.** You will need to plan and set aside time for shopping, preparation, and consumption of meals. Ideally, you will need two shopping days per week. Decide which these are now, and in this way you will have a good supply of fresh vegetables and fruit, an essential part of the diet. If you really can only go shopping once a week, you will have to store all your fruit and vegetables in the refrigerator or somewhere cool to prevent them from spoiling. This is particularly true during the warmer months of the year.

- **Go shopping before beginning your diet.** Supermarkets, as well as health food shops, have a wide range of the necessary foods. Rice-cakes and low-fat polyunsaturated margarine will be advisable for most people.

- **When you go shopping, go with your shopping list and stick to it.** Don't try to remember what to buy when you are in the supermarket. The presentation of foods in the supermarket is designed to stimulate your appetite, not your memory.

- **Go shopping after you have eaten, not before.** Letting someone who is hungry and overweight, and who hasn't eaten for six hours, loose in a supermarket should be a criminal offence! During the week, we suggest that you go shopping after breakfast or lunch, or perhaps after your evening meal. During the weekend, go shopping on Saturday after breakfast. If you have to do a major shop without having had a meal, eat one of your snacks first.

- **Eat regularly, at least three meals a day,** preferably with two small snacks. Never miss meals. Irregular eating leads to less healthy weight loss, and an increased feeling of hunger.

- **Eat from a small plate, not a large one.** A well-stocked medium sized lunch or breakfast plate looks more satisfying than a large dinner plate that is only half-filled.

- **Eating is an experience in its own right.** Make it one. Firstly, set aside time for preparing the meal. Always eat sitting down, and only sit down to eat when everything is ready: the meal itself, drink, cutlery, condiments. Do not listen

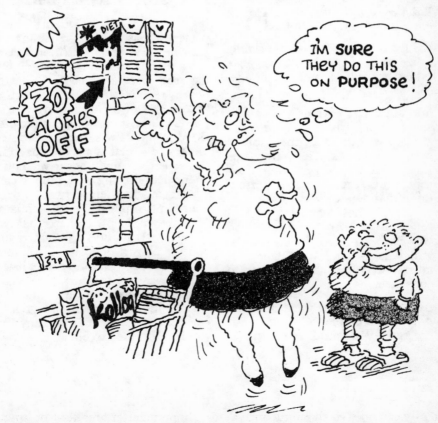

to the radio or watch the television while eating. Look at your food. Try to eat in company. The company of your own family, partner, or friends will help you to maintain self-discipline, and increase your enjoyment of eating.

- **Savour the flavour** of each mouthful, and chew your food well. Stop and try to detect the sensations in taste of each type of food that you are chewing.

- **Eat a wide variety of foods.** Do not eat a lot of one type of food.

- **Eat fresh foods whenever possible.** Frozen is acceptable if fresh vegetables or meat are not obtainable.

- **Never eat your meals in a hurry.** You are better eating just a small snack than hurrying a main meal. A good way to break the habit of eating too quickly is to put your knife and fork down after each mouthful. A return to the formal table manners of Victorian times may be the best way to stop us all eating in a hurry. Another good way is to say grace before meals, which is another way of appreciating what we are about to consume.

- **Always prepare one meal at a time** if at all possible. If this is not practical, you could try cooking a chicken to eat cold over several days; but once it is cooked, divide it up into the meal portions you require, and place them in the freezer or refrigerator as appropriate.

- **Use non-stick, iron, stainless steel, enamel or glass cookware.**

- **Avoid physical contact with prohibited foods,** e.g. when preparing foods for others.

DECISIONS TO LIVE BY

It is important to identify your personal reasons for wanting to be slimmer and feel healthier. Recent research has shown that people who list the consequences of dieting, positive and negative, and remind themselves of them regularly during the day, do twice as well on their diets as those people who just have routine dietary advice. It is a good idea to list the positive and negative consequences of dieting on an index card, which you can then carry around and refer to prior to eating, or exercising.

An example of a chart that you could construct on a card, or in your diary is shown opposite. Give some thought to each column before listing the reasons you want to lose weight. Complete it after eating – not before.

Once the chart is complete, refer to it at least at meal-times, and any time you feel tempted to cheat!

IMMEDIATE CONSEQUENCES

	Positive	Negative
Following the Vitality Diet	Improved mood Feeling of well-being Self-satisfaction Approval from friends and family Weight loss	Bother of educating oneself Possible withdrawal symptoms Changing old habits Having to change lifestyle Family eating habits change Having to exercise
Continuing with previous eating habits	No changes required Short-term satisfaction No expense on new clothes	Poor self-image Feel bloated and overweight Feel generally below par

LONG-TERM CONSEQUENCES

	Positive	Negative
Following the Vitality Diet	Feeling of well-being Pleasing appearance Sense of achievement Improved health for all the family	Not able to indulge in all your favourite foods and drinks
Continuing with previous eating habits	No effort required Social satisfaction of 'free' eating	Self-conscious of size Feel uncomfortable and bloated Feel unwell Increased health risks Expense of larger clothes!

18
The basic guidelines

Now let us look at the diet. It is probably similar in many ways to diets you have seen or read about before, but there are some very important differences.

STAGE I

This will provide, per day:

- 1,000–1,500 calories per day, depending on your needs
- 65 or more grams of protein
- 25 or more grams of fibre
- a good balance of vitamins and minerals.

This diet is relatively high in protein and fibre, and is very nutritious.

The first stage of the programme is designed to get you on to a balanced, low-calorie diet, and to cleanse your system so that in Stage II you will be able to tell which foods suit your body the most. There is a suggested menu for each day of the four weeks with guidelines for you to follow. You can adapt the menus for eating away from home, i.e. at work or even in a restaurant. Eating out will be the most difficult for the first two stages,

but you can certainly get away with it from time to time. There are packed lunch menus on page 151.

HOW TO WORK OUT YOUR CALORIE REQUIREMENTS

For women who wish to lose weight quickly and who are not physically active, an intake of 1,000 calories per day should be sufficient.

Most men should have 1,500 calories per day (and even more if physically active) as part of this weight-loss programme.

The menus are presented as a 1,000 calorie diet. If you feel when you read each day's diet that you will need more to eat, then you can increase the amount quite easily. By increasing the portion sizes by 25 per cent (a quarter), you will then have a 1,250 calorie intake per day. By increasing the portion sizes by 50 per cent (a half) you will bring your calorie intake up to 1,500 calories per day. In this way the diet is easy to adjust to your own requirements. If you do increase your calorie intake, ensure that you increase *all* the portions of *all* the foods and not just some, so that the nutritious balance of the diet will be maintained.

FOODS THAT CAN BE EATEN

In the first four weeks during Stage I, it is very important to eat only the allowed foods. If you introduce other foods you will lose the beneficial effects of the diet and it will be necessary for you to begin again!

✓ Meat and poultry

All meat, including lamb, beef, pork, chicken, turkey, other poultry and game, and offal, such as liver, kidneys, sweetbreads and hearts, can be eaten if desired. Meat and poultry can be fresh or frozen.

Meat must be lean, with all visible fat trimmed before cooking. Do not eat the skin of chicken or other poultry; it should be removed before or after cooking.

✓ Fish and shellfish

All types are included and they may be fresh or frozen. Do not eat the skin of fish as it is high in fat and calories.

Note: all meat, poultry, and fish should be cooked by grilling, dry-roasting, steaming, baking, or stir-frying with low-fat ingredients, e.g. tomatoes or vegetables.

✓ All vegetables

You can and should eat large amounts of vegetables, especially green ones or salad foods daily. Your allowance will be detailed in the daily menus.

Root vegetables, e.g. potatoes and parsnips, are limited to 4–6oz (115–170g) per day. Beans and peas, which are protein-rich vegetables, are also included in moderate amounts.

✓ Fruits

All fruits are allowed, except dried fruits, glacé fruits, dates, figs, mangoes, and tinned fruits with sugar. Keep tinned fruits without sugar to a minimum also.

If you want to eat bananas (the world's most popular fruit), half of one is equal to a single fruit portion. Your fruit allowance amounts to *three pieces* of fruit per day. Fruit can either be eaten whole or as a fruit salad. There is a recipe for Fruit salad on page 146.

✓ Reduced-calorie foods

Fortunately, there are now many excellent calorie-reduced versions of such foods as salad dressings, mayonnaise, soups, and baked beans. There are also a few low-calorie convenience dinners that are allowed. We have incorporated some Findus Lean Cuisine dinners and some of the Heinz Weight Watchers dinners into the menus. Do remember to read labels carefully, though, while you are on a restricted diet.

✓ Vegetable oils and vegetable mayonnaise

A small amount of these are allowed

daily. You can have up to two tea-spoons of a low-fat polyunsaturate-rich margarine, such as Flora Light, per day. There are no fried foods on the diet (you didn't really expect them, did you?), but there are some stir-fry dishes and here you just wipe the inside of the pan or wok with a piece of kitchen roll dipped in sunflower or corn oil.

✓ Nuts and seeds

Peanuts, Brazil nuts, almonds, pistachios, cashews, sunflower seeds, and sesame seeds are very nutritious, but unfortunately high in calories. A few nuts or seeds occasionally, perhaps ½oz (15g) chopped up, may be used. They can help to liven up a salad or be used as a nutritious snack, combined with an apple or another fruit.

✓ Rice and other salads

White or brown rice of any variety — long-grain, short-grain or basmati — is allowed. It will often be used instead of potatoes. Rice-cakes (a rice crispbread) can be used in place of bread. Additionally, buckwheat, bamboo shoots, millet, sago and tapioca can be used from time to time, but these are not usually very popular.

✓ Breakfast cereals

Only cornflakes and Rice Krispies are included in Stage I. They contain a good amount of protein and are fortified with extra vitamin B and iron. Other breakfast cereals are *not* allowed.

✓ Eggs

Up to seven eggs per week are allowed, unless you are known to have a very high cholesterol level. They are highly nutritious and very good value for money.

FOODS TO BE AVOIDED OR SEVERELY LIMITED

✗ Wheat, oat, barley, and rye

All foods made with these, apart from the exceptions given below, are to be avoided. This means no cakes, biscuits, puddings, pasta, pastry, pies, porridge, or breakfast cereals (apart from cornflakes or Rice Krispies). Bread is severely limited to two slices of white low-calorie bread, e.g. Slimcea.

✗ Dairy products

Cream and cheese are forbidden — even low-fat cottage cheese is out. Your milk allowance is very low, only 3 fluid ounces per day of skimmed milk, 1 pint (20floz/570ml) per week. You can use dried skimmed milk instead, or low-fat plain yogurt.

Butter or a polyunsaturated low-fat spread is allowed: one or two level teaspoonsful per day. However, if you have premenstrual tension, painful breasts, or an elevated blood cholesterol level, you should have a low-fat polyunsaturated spread instead of butter.

Foods containing milk, cream, cheese, milk solids, non-fat milk solids, lactalbumin, whey, caseinates, and lactose should be avoided. The only exception to this is poly-unsaturated margarine which often contains a very small amount of milk protein, lactalbumin or whey.

✘ Animal fats and some vegetable fats

Animal fats, some vegetable fats, hard margarines, lard, dripping and suet are out, as are palm oil and coconut oil, and foods containing them. Chemically, these vegetable oils are much more like saturated animal fats than good quality sunflower or corn oil which are high in the healthier polyunsaturates. Hard margarines which are made from hydrogenated vegetable oils are also off the menu.

✘ Sugar, honey, glucose, and fructose (fruit sugar)

Any food made with these should be avoided in the main. This means cakes, biscuits, most ice-cream, sweets of all kinds, chocolate, and puddings. This is not as depressing as it sounds. You will find that we have provided suggestions for low-calorie desserts for each evening of the diet.

We must stress the importance of reading the labels carefully before purchasing sweet food. Weight Watchers produce very good ice-cream, so hunt around until you find

what you need.

Fruit juices are high in fructose, which weight for weight has the same calories as sucrose (ordinary sugar). Leave the large helpings of honey for the bees!

✘ Alcoholic beverages

You name it — alcohol's out. Sorry! Don't do this diet over Christmas. Even low-calorie alcoholic drinks, though they are a great improvement, are all too high in calories. You will, however, get the chance to try out alcohol in the third week of Stage II of the diet.

✘ Yeast-rich foods

This includes any foods containing yeast extract: Marmite, Oxo, Knorr and other stock cubes, vinegar, any pickled food, chutneys, piccalilli, sauces, or condiments containing yeast extract or vinegar.

✘ Salt

Salt should not be used in cooking or at the table. This is particularly true if you experience fluid retention or high blood pressure. Salty foods such as ham, bacon and any other salted meats should be eaten sparingly. Crisps, peanuts and many conven-ience dinners are not on the menu at all. If you really cannot do without salt, then use a very small amount only. Put it on the side of your plate. Try flavouring any salads, vegetables, or cooked main dishes with pepper or herbs instead of salt. You should find that your taste for salt becomes less as you progress through the diet programme.

✘ Foods with additives

These cannot be avoided completely, but it is best to avoid those with some types of colouring and preservatives which can cause asthma, nettle-rash (urticaria), eczema, and possibly migraine.

Avoid the following additives where possible:

E102	Tartrazine
E104	Quinoline Yellow
E110	Sunset Yellow FCF or Orange Yellow
E122	Carmoisine or Azorubine
E123	Amaranth
E124	Ponceau 4R or Cochineal Red A
E127	Erythrosine BS
E131	Patent Blue V
E132	Indigo Carmine or Indigotine
E142	Green S or Acid Brilliant Green BS or Lissamine Green
E151	Black PN or Brilliant Black PN
E180	Pigment Rubine or Lithol Rubine BK
E220-	Sulphites — these may
227	worsen asthma in very sensitive individuals.

Other colourings are not likely to cause any adverse reactions.

✘ Suspect foods

Avoid any foods that you know or suspect do not suit you. For example, many people find some fruits, such as oranges or pineapple, too acidic. Even though they are not particularly high in calories you should avoid them. A not-infrequent problem is inability to digest beans, peas and some vegetables properly, resulting in excessive wind. Possible vegetables in this group include cabbage, cauliflower, onions, and sweetcorn. At this point, trust your own knowledge and experience. After all, it is this that we want to increase, so let's not go against anything you know already. Accordingly you may have to adapt the day's menu or recipes to suit yourself.

MODIFICATIONS

Vegetarians/vegans should also allow peas, beans, lentils, soya milk, non-fermented soya produce, and increased amounts of nuts, seeds and rice.

SYMPTOMS

You may notice during the beginning of Stage I that you experience some withdrawal symptoms as a direct result of giving up certain foods and drinks that you usually consume. These symptoms may be anything from headaches to fatigue or even depression. This will depend on your existing diet. For example, if you are consuming lots of cups of coffee or tea, cola drinks, or refined sweet foods, you may find the first week of the diet is quite a challenge!

It is probably best to begin the diet when you have a quiet week to spare. A word of advice to women of child-bearing age is to begin the diet just after your period has arrived and not in the week your period is due. The reason for this is to prevent additional symptoms occurring at a time when you might be suffering from PMT.

You will need the time to orient yourself to your new way of eating and to get plenty of relaxation. This doesn't mean that you should take time off work; quite the opposite, as it is preferable that you remain occupied while on the diet. Just keep social engagements that involve eating to a minimum. Then, if you feel tired or experience any with-drawal symptoms, you can go off to rest without any guilty feelings of having let others down.

After the first week or so of follow-ing the diet, with any possible withdrawal symptoms behind you, things should look up. By Week 3, you should have lost a few pounds — at least four, possibly as many as eight — and you may notice that a number of minor health problems have begun to improve. By Week 4, you should be feeling quite well, perhaps better than you have felt for some time and, with any luck, you will be a good deal nearer to your target weight.

STAGE II

You start becoming a 'nutritional detective' during the second four-week period: trying out groups of foods to see whether they push your weight back up or produce other unwanted symptoms or side-effects.

For each week there are different instructions. You will need to follow these very carefully as this is an important stage of the diet. If you follow the instructions precisely, you will end up with a diet that is really tailored to suit your own body.

You may experience some symp-toms or 'side-effects' from the foods under test. These should pass off within two or three days. There are a large number of symptoms that could be experienced, but these should only be those that cleared up in Stage I. They include migraine, headaches, eczema, nettle-rash (urticaria), rhi-nitis, asthma, abdominal bloating and discomfort, constipation, diarr-hoea, wind, anxiety, irritability, insomnia, and possibly premenstrual tension. If and when you do have a reaction to individual food groups, you may feel that you have had a setback. On the contrary, any re-action should be regarded as a positive step. It means that you have dis-covered some foods that don't really suit your body at the moment. Any reaction, should it occur, should not be worse than those you have already experienced, and is likely to last no more than three days. If you do exper-ience a reaction, you will need to stop eating the foods that are causing the problem. You will find instructions on how to go about this in Stage II.

Daily diaries

It is vital to make sure that you

complete the daily diaries during each stage. You will need these as you go along, so do ensure you keep accurate records.

STAGE III

During the final two-week period you will be eating a diet composed of the foods you have selected through trial and error in the preceding four weeks. You should continue to lose weight and to feel more and more healthy as the weeks go by.

You will have gained the knowledge of how to tell when a particular food does not suit your body and how to deal with any bloating or other symptoms that may occur as a result. If you have lost enough weight, you will be able to increase your calorie intake by 20–40 per cent. By that stage, you should feel totally at home with your new diet and confident that you can maintain it as a lifestyle with ease in the place of your former diet.

19
Stage I — the first four weeks

So now you are ready to begin. Make sure you read the instructions carefully and only begin when you are satisfied that you have a good understanding of what is needed. For the next four weeks you will need to follow the diet outlined as closely as you possibly can. There is a page set aside for each day which consists of the following:

- your daily diet sheet
- some key facts
- a weight and symptom chart.

DAILY DIET SHEET
For each day of the diet we have devised a specific menu to follow, which amounts to approximately 1,000 calories per day. The daily recommendations are fairly basic. We have tried to keep them simple to prepare, bearing in mind that most of us are busy and therefore prefer to spend the minimum time possible preparing food.

If you like cooking and have the time to experiment, there is a recipe section on pages 133–150, which you might like to try, and in the reading list you will find a selection of recipe books that you might like to dip into. You may prefer to keep the diet simple during your working week and to save the more elaborate meals for the weekends or, if you feel really adventurous, for dinner parties. Unless you absolutely hate cooking, or are just too busy, it is preferable that you experiment with some of the recipes in order to keep the diet interesting. It really is not necessary to get bored with eating the same foods over and over during the next four weeks.

The main point to understand is that the diet is flexible, *but* you must:

- stick to 1,000 calories per day (unless you have chosen to increase your calorie allowance)
- eat only the foods allowable in the stage you are currently on.

FACTS
- There is much important information relating to diet and lifestyle, of which you may not be aware. So there are two or more key facts each day for your education.

All the facts are interesting; some may come as quite a surprise, while others may not.

Apart from being slimmer and healthier at the end of the diet, you should also be quite knowledgeable on the subject of diet in general, and be your own expert on the diet that's right for you.

WEIGHT AND SYMPTOM CHART

At the foot of the page for each day you will see a little weight and symptom chart. We have provided this so that you can keep a daily record of your progress on the diet and of your weight.

Make sure you weigh yourself daily, preferably at a similar time each day and in a similar state of dress or undress. For example, you could try to get into a routine of weighing yourself first thing in the morning before you get dressed. Don't forget to make your chart for each day as you go along. It's not wise to rely on your memory, which may not be quite so accurate.

You will also need to complete the symptom section of the chart on a daily basis. Mark in any symptoms that you have experienced on *that day only*. On any day that you are symptom-free, just mark in 'no symptoms'.

MAKING A START

A shopping list

Read through the diet section for the first four weeks and read through the recipes if you are likely to be using them. Then with a *full stomach after a meal* make yourself a shopping list, and go shopping. Most of the foods suggested will fit into a moderate budget. Some foods, however, are seasonal, so when it comes to buying fruit, vegetables and salad, for example, you will need to look out for those products that are in plentiful supply at the time, and consequently more reasonably priced.

A DIET TO SUIT YOUR LIFESTYLE

Although we have prepared suggested menus for each day, it is important to stress that these meals are flexible as long as you stick to the suggested foods for each week and the calorie allowance per day.

If you prefer to select your own meals, rather than follow our suggestion for the day, you will find selections of breakfasts, salads and snacks to choose from, with precise calorie values for each, on pages 99–100, and main meal recipes at the end of Stage I and each week of Stage II. Do not forget to weigh your food to get the portion sizes right.

Breakfast

We have suggested a variety of breakfasts to keep the menus interesting and to demonstrate the variety possible on this diet. We do, however, appreciate that being creatures of habit, many people may prefer to have a similar breakfast each day, for the sake of speed and perhaps taste also. While fruit and cereals may seem appealing to some of us for breakfast, others may prefer fish or even bacon and tomatoes.

Lunches

If you are out of your home at lunch-time, you will need to keep lunch as simple as possible. On page 151, you will find a selection of packed lunches which we hope you will agree are relatively portable.

Desserts

We have planned the desserts to follow on from the evening meal, as after the main meal we often like to have something sweet to eat. How-ever, if you happen to be in a situation where you are out for lunch, then you can happily have your dessert at lunch-time instead of that evening. On pages 146–150, there is a selection of desserts you can choose from during the four weeks of Stage I.

Snacks

You will probably feel better if you eat little and often, as this helps to maintain your blood sugar level, and prevents you from getting 'the munchies', especially during the first four weeks of the diet, when you are first restricting your diet.

Beverages

You can drink water freely during the course of the diet. Apart from that you have an allowance of the following:

- 1 or 2 cups of black tea or coffee per day (except during Week 4 of Stage II, when you may be drinking more)
- 1 small (4floz/115ml) glass of orange juice, or 2 small glasses of tomato juice per day
- Herb tea (without milk) whenever you desire it.

SUMMARIES

To help you work out your own menus, here are summaries of the salads and the foods that go to make up breakfasts and snacks. You can avoid any foods you do not like and replace them with others from these lists so long as you do not exceed your daily calorie allowance.

Breakfasts	Calories
2 boiled eggs	160
2 scrambled eggs	160
4oz (115g) poached mushrooms	14
2 grilled tomatoes	16
1 slice lean bacon, grilled	80
1 slice slimmer's bread	40
1 rice-cake	28
1oz Rice Krispies	105
1oz (30g) cornflakes	104
½ grapefruit	17
Fruit salad	100
Fruit	50
3½oz (100g) yogurt	40
1 tablespoon linseeds	10
1 teaspoon butter	50

1 teaspoon low-calorie
  margarine 25
3floz (85ml) skimmed milk 28
Glass of orange juice 50
Black tea 0
Black coffee 0

Snacks | Calories

	Calories
1 piece of fresh fruit (but ½ banana)	50
2oz (55g) raw carrot	13
6oz (170g) celery sticks	12
1 rice-cake	28
1 slice of slimmer's bread	40
1 teaspoon low-calorie jam	10
½ portion rice salad	55
1 portion of any other salad (see list)	

Salads | Calories

Salads	Calories
Beansprout	65
Bean and sweetcorn	25
Beetroot and cabbage	47
Cauliflower and carrot	30
Cole-slaw	40
Courgette and cauliflower	27
Fruity cabbage	75
Ginger and carrot	36
Green	32
Root	31
Summer	45
Tomato and celery	20
Vegetable	50
Bean	110
Brown rice	110
Potato	125

(see pages 142-145
for recipes)

STAGE 1 — MENUS

Foods marked with an asterisk (*) are included in the recipe section on pages 133–150.

WEEK 1 — DAY 1

Breakfast	Calories
2 boiled eggs (size 3)	160
2 rice-cakes/1 slice slimmer's toast	56
1 teaspoon (5ml) low-calorie margarine	25

Mid-morning snack

3½oz (100g) low-calorie yogurt	40
1 chopped apple	50

Lunch

5oz (140g) canned salmon	218
*Beansprout salad	65

Mid-afternoon snack

2oz (55g) raw carrot	13
3oz (85g) stick celery	6

Dinner

*Cumin chicken	145
4oz (115g) broccoli	20
4oz (115g) carrots	21
4oz (115g) potatoes	90

Dessert

Fruit salad	100
TOTAL CALORIES	**1,009**

FACTS

- A calorie is a unit of energy and each food provides a certain amount of energy when it is 'burnt' or metabolized by the body.

- A calorie is actually a tiny amount of energy. When we say a food contains so many 'calories' we really mean kilo-calories or thousand calories. So an apple contains 50–60 kilocalories, not 50–60 calories.

So, welcome to your 1,000 kilo-calorie (1,000,000 calorie) diet!

Daily chart

Starting weight _____

Symptoms _____

_____

_____

_____

_____

_____

WEEK 1 — DAY 2

Breakfast	Calories
1oz (30g) Rice Krispies	105
3floz (85ml) skimmed milk	28
1 apple (chopped into Rice Krispies)	50
1 tablespoon linseeds (e.g. Linusit Gold) sprinkled on top	10

Mid-morning snack

2oz (55g) raw carrot	13
3oz (85g) stick celery	6

Lunch

4oz (115g) lean ham	135
*Fruity cabbage salad	75
4oz (115g) jacket potato	96
1 tablespoon (15ml) low-calorie dressing	25

Mid-afternoon snack

1 piece of fruit	50

Dinner

*Liver with orange	250
4oz (115g) cauliflower	10
4oz (115g) French beans	8
2oz (55g) brown rice	66

Dessert

*Gooseberry jelly	70
TOTAL CALORIES	997

FACTS

● Different foods have different calorie values for the same weight. Water and fibre in food provide no calories at all, so vegetables and salad foods which are high in both water and fibre are low in calories.

● Fats contain more than twice the amount of calories as carbohydrates or proteins for the same weight.

Daily chart

Today's weight _____

Symptoms _____

_____

_____

_____

_____

_____

WEEK 1 — DAY 3

Breakfast	Calories
½ grapefruit (6oz/170g)	17
1 scrambled egg (size 3)	80
2 medium tomatoes (4oz/115g)	16
2 rice-cakes or 1 slice slimmer's bread	56

Mid-morning snack

4oz (115g) raw carrots	26
3oz (85g) stick celery	6

Lunch

5oz (140g) sardines in tomato sauce, tinned or fresh	250
4oz (115g) jacket potato	96
*Green salad	32

Mid-afternoon snack

1 piece of fruit	50

Dinner

*Pork with pineapple sauce	220
2oz (55g) brown rice	66
4oz (115g) broccoli	20
4oz (115g) cabbage	10

Dessert

*Cranberry sorbet	50
TOTAL CALORIES	995

FACTS

● An individual's calorie requirement varies with age, sex, physical activity and other health factors.

● To lose weight the intake of calories from the diet must be less than that required – so that the shortfall is made up by burning off some of the excess weight, which is mainly fatty tissue deposits.

Daily chart

Today's weight _____

Symptoms _____

_____

_____

_____

_____

_____

WEEK 1 — DAY 4

Breakfast	Calories
1oz (30g) cornflakes	104
3floz (85ml) skimmed milk	28

Mid-morning snack

1 rice-cake with 1 teaspoon (5ml) low-calorie jam	38
1 piece of fruit	50

Lunch

4oz (115g) cold chicken (breast)	140
2oz (55g) brown rice	66
*Vegetable salad	50
1 tablespoon (15ml) low-calorie salad dressing	25

Mid-afternoon snack

2oz (55g) raw carrot	13
6oz (170g) sticks of celery	12

Dinner

*Stuffed mackerel	250
4oz (115g) peas	59
4oz (115g) courgettes	11
4oz (115g) jacket potato	96

Dessert

*Jellied grapefruit	70

TOTAL CALORIES	1,012

FACTS

● The rate of weight loss is not influenced particularly by what form the calories are in. But if you do not take enough protein and just live on carbohydrates, e.g. an all-fruit diet, you will lose muscle tissue, rather than fat.

● Taking in too much protein will result in you putting on weight, as it can be converted to fat. It is a matter of getting the right balance of protein, carbohydrate and fat.

Daily chart

Today's weight _____

Symptoms _____

_____

_____

_____

_____

WEEK 1 — DAY 5

Breakfast	Calories
1 scrambled egg (size 3)	80
3oz (85g) red peppers and green peppers, chopped	12
2 rice-cakes/1 slice slimmer's bread	56
1 teaspoon (5ml) low-calorie margarine	25

Mid-morning snack

½ grated apple	25

Lunch

1 can Weight Watchers spring vegetable soup	65
*Tomato jacket	119
*Beansprout salad	65
4oz (115g) lettuce	14

Mid-afternoon snack

3½oz (100g) Shape yogurt	40

Dinner

4oz (115g) grilled lean lamb chops	222
4oz (115g) boiled potatoes	90
4oz (115g) sweetcorn, canned	85
4oz (115g) marrow	8

Dessert

*Peach sundae	95
TOTAL CALORIES	**1,001**

FACTS

● Getting the balance right means getting adequate amounts of the different vitamins and minerals that your body needs. Lack of them can produce a number of illnesses. This weight-loss diet is very carefully balanced to help minimize these problems.

● Taking more or extra vitamins will neither make you into Super-woman or Superman, nor speed your rate of weight loss. Some people on prolonged weight-loss diets will need a supplement to make sure that deficiencies do not develop.

Daily chart

Today's weight _____

Symptoms _____

_____

_____

_____

_____

_____

WEEK 1 — DAY 6

Breakfast	Calories
1 rasher lean bacon (1¼oz/35g)	80
2 grilled tomatoes	16
2 rice-cakes or 1 slice slimmer's bread	56
1 teaspoon (5ml) low-calorie spread	25

Mid-morning snack

3½oz (100g) Shape yogurt	40
½ grated apple	25

Lunch

5oz (140g) fresh plaice, grilled	131
4oz (115g) jacket potato	96
*Courgette and cauliflower salad	27
4oz (115g) lettuce	14
1 tablespoon (15ml) low-calorie dressing	25

Mid-afternoon snack

1 rice-cake	28
1 teaspoon (5ml) low-calorie jam	10
½ apple	25

Dinner

*Chicken paprika	220
2oz (55g) brown rice	66
4oz (115g) spinach	34
4oz (115g) cauliflower	10

Dessert

*Baked apple	80
TOTAL CALORIES	**1,008**

FACTS

● There are two sorts of vitamins: some are soluble in fat (vitamins A, D, E and K), and some soluble in water (vitamins B and C).

● Vitamins, unlike proteins and calories, are required in only tiny amounts, fractions of a gram per day. They are needed to help along important steps in the body's metabolism, influencing growth, producing energy, controlling hormones, helping resistance to infection, and maintaining the health of all the tissues in the body.

Daily chart

Today's weight _____

Symptoms _____

_____

_____

_____

_____

_____

WEEK 1 — DAY 7

Breakfast	Calories
2 scrambled eggs	160
2 rice-cakes/1 slice slimmer's bread	56

Mid-morning snack

½ grated apple and 3½oz (100g) natural yogurt	65

Lunch

4oz (115g) grilled chicken breast	140
*Tomato sauce	35
2oz (55g) boiled brown rice	66
4oz (115g) cauliflower	10
4oz (115g) broccoli	20

Mid-afternoon snack

3oz (85g) stick celery	6
1 piece of fruit	50

Dinner

4oz (115g) roast lamb, lean only	196
4oz (115g) baked potato	96
4oz (115g) French beans	8
4oz (115g) carrots	21

Dessert

*Jellied grapefruit	70
TOTAL CALORIES	999

FACTS

● Deficiency of fat-soluble vitamins is quite rare, as the body stores them in the liver and other organs. You would have to eat a very poor diet, lose a lot of weight, or be very ill for any serious deficiency to occur.

● The water-soluble vitamins, however, are not usually stored in the body in any great amount, so deficiency can develop within a few weeks or months if the diet is poor.

Daily chart

Today's weight _____

Symptoms _____

_____

_____

_____

_____

WEEK-ENDING CHART
Stage I

Date

Total weight change this week	Withdrawal symptoms experienced	General degree of well-being*	Any other comments or observations
Weight at beginning of week			
Weight at end of week			
Total weight loss			

*Score degree of well-being
Very well 3   Well 2   Fair 1   Unwell 0

WEEK 2 — DAY 1

Breakfast	Calories
1oz (30g) cornflakes	104
3floz (85ml) skimmed milk	28
1 chopped apple	50

Mid-morning snack

2 rice-cakes with 2 teaspoons low-calorie jam	76

Lunch

5oz (140g) sardines in tomato sauce	250
4oz (115g) jacket potato	96
*Root salad	31
4oz (115g) lettuce	14
1 tablespoon (15ml) low-calorie salad dressing	25

Mid-afternoon snack

4oz (115g) raw carrots	26
3oz (85g) stick celery	6

Dinner

*Vegetable curry	185
2oz (55g) brown rice	66

Dessert

*Cranberry sorbet or fresh fruit	50
TOTAL CALORIES	1,007

FACTS

● Animal vitamin A, retinol, and vegetable vitamin A, beta-carotene, are needed for healthy eyes, good vision in the dark, healthy skin, and adequate resistance to infection.

● The best dietary sources of vitamin A are liver, carrots, milk, eggs, butter, margarine, and all yellow/green vegetables and fruits.

Daily chart

Today's weight _____

Symptoms _____

_____

_____

_____

_____

_____

WEEK 2 — DAY 2

Breakfast	Calories
2 boiled eggs	160
2 rice-cakes/1 slice slimmer's bread	56
1 teaspoon low-calorie jam	10
1 teaspoon low-calorie margarine	25

Mid-morning snack
1 piece of fruit	50

Lunch
5oz (140g) steamed trout	125
*Ginger and carrot salad	36
4oz (115g) lettuce	14
4oz (115g) jacket potato	96

Mid-afternoon snack
2oz (55g) raw carrot	13
6oz (170g) sticks celery	12

Dinner
*Liver kebabs	225
2oz (55g) brown rice	66
2oz (55g) sweetcorn	43

Dessert
*Gooseberry jelly	70

TOTAL CALORIES	1,001

FACTS

● Vitamin D is not really a vitamin! It's a hormone that is produced in the body as a result of skin exposure to sunlight. As a hormone it stimulates the absorption of calcium from the food we have eaten and the healthy development of teeth and bones.

● The reason vitamin D was regarded as a vitamin is because it is found in our food, and this is important for those who do not receive adequate exposure to sunlight — for example, the housebound elderly. Good sources of vitamin D in the diet are butter, margarine, milk, eggs, fish, and fish liver oil.

Daily chart

Today's weight _____

Symptoms _____

_____

_____

_____

_____

WEEK 2 — DAY 3

Breakfast	Calories
1oz (30g) cornflakes	104
1 piece of fruit, chopped	50
3floz (95ml) milk	28

Mid-morning break

1 rice-cake	28
1 teaspoon low-calorie jam	10

Lunch

4oz (115g) tongue, cooked	240
*Tomato and celery salad	20
4oz (115g) lettuce	14
2oz (55g) brown rice	66

Mid-afternoon snack

1 piece of fruit	50

Dinner

*Haddock parcels	180
4oz (115g) marrow	8
4oz (115g) carrots	21
4oz (115g) potatoes	90

Dessert

*Peach sundae	95

TOTAL CALORIES	1,004

FACTS

● Vitamin E is really a group of plant oils called tocopherols. They have the unique ability to prevent the deterioration that occurs in certain fats as a result of exposure to oxygen in the air, and so help to prevent deterioration of fats in the body. This is needed for healthy skin and nervous system function.

● Though deficiency is very rare indeed, you can ensure a good supply of vitamin E by eating nuts, seeds and their oils, green vegetables, and wholegrains.

Daily chart

Today's weight _____

Symptoms _____

_____

_____

_____

_____

_____

WEEK 2 — DAY 4

Breakfast	Calories
2 pieces of fruit, chopped	100
with 3½oz (100g) Shape yogurt	40
1 tablespoon linseeds (e.g. Linusit Gold)	10

Mid-morning snack

2 rice-cakes	56
2 teaspoons low-calorie jam	20

Lunch

*Orange and carrot soup	55
4oz (115g) jacket potato	96
*Bean salad	110
4oz (115g) lettuce	14

Mid-afternoon snack

4oz (115g) raw carrots	26
6oz (170g) sticks celery	12

Dinner

*Lamb and aubergine bake	260
4oz (115g) leeks	27
4oz (115g) cauliflower	10
4oz (115g) mashed potatoes, with	90
1floz (30ml) milk	9

Dessert

*Fruit snow	70

TOTAL CALORIES	1,005

FACTS

● Vitamin K, the last of the fat-soluble vitamins, is needed for the body to heal cuts and bruises. Deficiency results in excessive bleeding or bruising after even minor accidents or injuries.

● Again, deficiency is rare and occurs only in very ill people, new-born children, or those on prolonged courses of antibiotics.

Daily chart

Today's weight _____

Symptoms _____

_____

_____

_____

_____

_____

WEEK 2 — DAY 5

Breakfast	Calories
2 boiled eggs	160
2 rice-cakes/1 slice slimmer's bread	56

Mid-morning snack
4oz (115g) raw carrot	26
6oz (170g) sticks celery	12

Lunch
5oz (140g) grilled cod	134
4oz (115g) boiled potatoes	90
4oz (115g) carrots	21
4oz (115g) peas	59

Mid-afternoon snack
1 rice-cake	28
1 teaspoon low-calorie jam	10

Dinner
4oz (115g) grilled sirloin steak/rump steak	192
*Tomato sauce	35
4oz (115g) jacket potato	96
4oz (115g) French beans	8
4oz (115g) broccoli	20

Dessert
*Cranberry sorbet or 1 piece of fruit	50
TOTAL CALORIES	**997**

FACTS

● The water-soluble B vitamins contain several different types: vitamin B_1 (thiamine), B_2 (riboflavin), B_3 (nicotinic acid), B_5 (pantothenic acid), B_6 (pyridoxine), B_{12} (cobalamin), and folic acid.

● The worst enemy of B vitamins is alcohol — consuming more than 2 units per day for women, or 3 units a day for men, puts them at risk. Smokers also have lower levels of some B vitamins.

Daily chart

Today's weight _____

Symptoms _____

_____

_____

_____

_____

WEEK 2 — DAY 6

Breakfast	Calories
1oz (30g) Rice Krispies	105
1 chopped apple	50
3floz (85ml) skimmed milk	28

Mid-morning snack

2 rice-cakes with 2 teaspoons low-calorie jam	76

Lunch

2 egg omelette with	160
2oz (55g) peppers	8
2oz (55g) sweetcorn, canned	43

Mid-afternoon snack

1 piece of fruit	50

Dinner

*Prawn and vegetable stir-fry	225
3oz (85g) brown rice, with	99
1oz (30g) hazelnuts	95

Dessert

*Jellied grapefruit	70

TOTAL CALORIES	1,009

FACTS

● Vitamin B$_1$ (thiamine), is needed for healthy nerves and muscles. Good food sources are wheat, other grains, pork, other meats, peas, beans, and nuts. Deficiency is particularly likely in moderate to heavy alcohol consumers, the elderly, and those with mental problems.

● Deficiency can produce poor memory, mental deterioration, mood changes, painful weak muscles, and nerve and heart damage.

Daily chart

Today's weight _____

Symptoms _____

_____

_____

_____

_____

WEEK 2 — DAY 7

Breakfast	Calories
½ grapefruit (6oz/170g)	17
1 rasher lean bacon (1¼oz/35g)	80
2 grilled tomatoes (4oz/115g)	16
1 slice slimmer's bread	40

Mid-morning snack

1 piece of fruit	50

Lunch

1 can Weight Watchers beef and vegetable soup	75
4oz (115g) jacket potato	96
5oz (140g) sardines in tomato sauce	250

Mid-afternoon snack

1 rice-cake	28
1 teaspoon low-calorie jam	10

Dinner

4oz (115g) roast chicken breast	167
4oz (115g) boiled potatoes	90
4oz (115g) cabbage	10
4oz (115g) turnips	16

Dessert

*Rhubarb and ginger mousse	50
TOTAL CALORIES	**995**

FACTS

● Deficiency of vitamins B_2 (riboflavin), B_3 (nicotinic acid), or B_5 (pantothenic acid) is not common. They are all needed for energy, fat, or protein metabolism. Good sources are dairy products, meat, fish, beans, peas, and grains.

● A deficiency could produce cracking or peeling of the lips, a sore tongue, depression and mood changes, but this is likely only in the elderly, heavy alcohol consumers, and those on a prolonged weight-loss diet.

Daily chart

Today's weight _____

Symptoms _____

_____

_____

_____

_____

WEEK-ENDING CHART
Stage I

Date			
Total weight change this week	Withdrawal symptoms experienced	General degree of well-being*	Any other comments or observations
Weight at beginning of week			
Weight at end of week			
Total weight loss			

*Score degree of well-being
Very well 3　　　Well 2　　　Fair 1　　　Unwell 0

WEEK 3 — DAY 1

Breakfast	Calories
1oz (30g) Rice Krispies	105
3floz (85ml) skimmed milk	28
1 grated apple	50

Mid-morning snack

2oz (55g) raw carrot	13
3oz (85g) stick of celery	6

Lunch

1 can of Weight Watchers tomato soup	75
*Bean salad	110
*Green salad	32
2oz (55g) cooked weight brown rice	66

Afternoon snack

1 piece of fruit	50

Dinner

*Kidney casserole	270
4oz (115g) boiled potatoes	90
4oz (115g) Brussels sprouts	20
2oz (55g) sweetcorn	43

Dessert

1 piece of fresh fruit	50

TOTAL CALORIES	1,008

FACTS

● Vitamin B_6 (pyridoxine) is essential for protein metabolism and the production of brain chemicals that affect mood and mental function. Good sources of B_6 include beef, chicken, nuts, cauliflower, potatoes, peas, bananas, and wheat.

● Mild deficiency of vitamin B_6 is not uncommon in the 'normal population', particularly in women and in smokers. It is not certain how important this is but it might influence mood, hormone function, and resistance to infection. It is obviously wise to ensure a good intake of this vitamin.

Daily chart

Today's weight _____

Symptoms _____

_____

_____

_____

_____

_____

WEEK 3 — DAY 2

Breakfast	Calories
2 pieces of fruit, chopped	100
3½oz (100g) Shape yogurt	40

Mid-morning snack

2 rice-cakes with 2 teaspoons low-calorie jam	76

Lunch

*Salmon with scrambled eggs	180
*Courgette and cauliflower salad	27
1 tablespoon (15ml) low-calorie dressing	25
4oz (115g) jacket potato	96

Mid-afternoon snack

1 apple	50

Dinner

*Pork with pineapple sauce	220
4oz (115g) French beans	8
4oz (115g) broccoli	20
4oz (115g) potatoes	90

Dessert

*Fruit snow	70

TOTAL CALORIES	1,002

FACTS

● Vitamin B_{12} and folic acid are needed to produce healthy red blood cells and to maintain the health of the nervous system. Good sources of vitamin B_{12} are all meats and other animal products, especially liver. Strict vegetarians and vegans are at risk of deficiency. Folic acid is plentiful in liver and all green leafy vegetables.

● Deficiency of either of these two vitamins can produce anaemia and nerve damage. Lack of folic acid in women in the first part of pregnancy increases the risk of the baby developing spina bifida — a serious defect of the nervous system.

Daily chart

Today's weight _____

Symptoms _____

_____

_____

_____

_____

WEEK 3 — DAY 3

Breakfast	Calories
1oz (30g) Rice Krispies	105
3floz (85ml) skimmed milk	28
1 chopped apple	50

Mid-morning snack

4oz (115g) raw carrots	26
6oz (170g) sticks of celery	12

Lunch

5oz (140g) raw weight grilled herring	225
*Beansprout salad	65
2oz (55g) brown rice	66

Mid-afternoon snack

1 rice-cake with 1 teaspoon (5ml) of low-calorie jam	38

Dinner

*Haddock Florentine	170
4oz (115g) carrots	21
4oz (115g) courgettes	11
4oz (115g) boiled potatoes	90

Dessert

*Peach sundae	95

TOTAL CALORIES	1,002

FACTS

● Vitamin C (ascorbic acid) is needed for healthy blood vessels and good tissue healing. Deficiency occurred during prolonged sailing voyages in the eighteenth century, when lack of fresh fruit and vegetables produced the condition of scurvy. Depression, poor appetite, bleeding gums, and poorly healing wounds were the main problems.

● Nowadays, vitamin C deficiency is rare. You would have to eat a very unhealthy diet indeed, avoiding all fresh fruit and vegetables. Smokers have lower levels of vitamin C and should take extra care with their diet — or better still, give up smoking.

Daily chart

Today's weight _____

Symptoms _____

_____

_____

_____

_____

WEEK 3 — DAY 4

Breakfast	Calories
2 poached eggs	160
2 grilled tomatoes	16
1 slice of slimmer's bread	40

Mid-morning snack

1 piece of fruit	50

Lunch

4oz (115g) of Weight Watchers spring vegetable soup	65
4oz (115g) jacket potato	96
8oz (225g) Weight Watchers baked beans	122
*Cole-slaw	40

Mid-afternoon snack

1 rice-cake with 1 teaspoon (5ml) low-calorie jam	38

Dinner

*Cumin chicken	145
4oz (115g) broccoli	20
4oz (115g) carrots	21
4oz (115g) potato	90

Dessert

Fruit salad	100

TOTAL CALORIES	1,003

FACTS

● The minerals can be divided into bulk minerals and trace minerals. Both sorts of minerals, like vitamins, are needed by the body for a normal healthy metabolism.

● Bulk minerals are needed in substantial amounts as they are used for the formation of the skeleton. They include: calcium, magnesium, phosphorus, sodium, potassium, and chlorine. There are several trace minerals and these serve very special functions.

Daily chart

Today's weight _____

Symptoms _____

_____

_____

_____

_____

_____

WEEK 3 — DAY 5

Breakfast	Calories
1oz (30g) cornflakes	104
3floz (85ml) skimmed milk	28
½ chopped apple	25

Mid-morning snack

1 rice-cake with 1 teaspoon (5ml) low-calorie jam	38

Lunch

5oz (140g) mackerel in tomato sauce or fresh grilled	194
2 medium tomatoes	16
4oz (115g) lettuce	14
4oz (115g) grated carrots	26
2oz (55g) brown rice	66

Mid-afternoon snack

2oz (55g) raw carrots	13

Dinner

4oz (115g) lamb chop, grilled	222
4oz (115g) boiled potatoes	90
4oz (115g) cabbage	10
4oz (115g) sweetcorn	86

Dessert

*Fruit snow	70

TOTAL CALORIES	1,002

FACTS

● Calcium is found in large amounts in all dairy products except butter, and in sardines, nuts, and green vegetables. Magnesium is plentiful in all green vegetables, wheat, other grains, nuts, seeds, and beans or peas. Both are needed for healthy bones, muscles, and nerves.

● In the long term, dietary adequacy is important. Calcium absorption is reduced by poor protein intake, bran, excessive amounts of wholemeal bread, coffee, or alcohol. Regular exercise greatly assists in the calcium being laid down as bone.

Daily chart

Today's weight _____

Symptoms _____

_____

_____

_____

_____

_____

WEEK 3 — DAY 6

Breakfast	Calories
2 scrambled eggs	160
2 grilled tomatoes (4oz/115g)	16
1 slice of slimmer's bread	40
1 teaspoon of low-calorie spread	25
1 teaspoon of low-calorie jam	10

Mid-morning snack

3½oz (100g) natural yogurt	40
1 grated apple	50

Lunch

5oz (140g) (raw weight) fresh plaice, grilled	105
4oz (115g) jacket potato	96
*Fruity cabbage salad	75
1 tablespoon (15ml) low-calorie dressing	25

Mid-afternoon snack

1 rice-cake with 1 teaspoon low-calorie jam	38

Dinner

*Vegetable curry	185
2oz (55g) brown rice	66

Dessert

*Jellied grapefruit	70
TOTAL CALORIES	**1,001**

FACTS

- Sodium and potassium are two similar minerals which act as opposites in the body. Large amounts of sodium are found outside the cells of the body, such as in the bloodstream, and most of the potassium is found inside the cells. The difference is needed for the proper function of all cells, especially the nervous system and muscles.

- A lack of potassium or sodium can cause muscle weakness. The best sources of potassium are vegetables and fruit. Most of our sodium comes as salt added to our food in preparation, cooking, or at the table. Too much salt can cause a rise in blood pressure or aggravate fluid retention.

Daily chart

Today's weight _____

Symptoms _____

_____

_____

_____

_____

_____

WEEK 3 — DAY 7

Breakfast	Calories
1 poached egg	80
1 rasher of lean bacon (1¼oz/35g)	80
1 grilled tomato (2oz/55g)	8
1 slice slimmer's bread	40

Mid-morning snack

1 piece of fresh fruit	50

Lunch

4oz (115g) lean ham	135
2oz (55g) lettuce	7
*Bean and sweetcorn salad	25
2oz (55g) brown rice	66

Mid-afternoon snack

4oz (15g) raw carrots	26

Dinner

*Stuffed mackerel	250
4oz (115g) peas	59
4oz (115g) courgettes	11
4oz (115g) jacket potato	96

Dessert

*Gooseberry jelly	70

TOTAL CALORIES	1,003

FACTS

● The trace minerals, like some vitamins, have very particular functions. Iron is needed for forming haemoglobin, the red pigment of the blood, and lack of it will cause anaemia. Iodine is needed for the function of the thyroid glands which control the metabolism. Zinc is needed for growth, healthy skin, and hormone production. Chromium is needed for good control of the blood sugar levels.

● The best way to get all your trace minerals is to eat a wide variety of foods from animal and vegetable sources, avoiding refined and processed foods.

Daily chart

Today's weight _____

Symptoms _____

_____

_____

_____

_____

_____

WEEK-ENDING CHART
Stage I

Date			
Total weight change this week	Withdrawal symptoms experienced	General degree of well-being*	Any other comments or observations
Weight at beginning of week			
Weight at end of week			
Total weight loss			

*Score degree of well-being
Very well 3   Well 2   Fair 1   Unwell 0

WEEK 4 — DAY 1

Breakfast	Calories
1oz (30g) cornflakes	104
3floz (85ml) skimmed milk	28

Mid-morning snack

2oz (55g) raw carrot	13
6oz (170g) sticks of celery	12

Lunch

5oz (140g) sardines in tomato sauce	250
Jacket potato	96
*Green salad	32
1 tablespoon (15ml) low-calorie dressing	25

Mid-afternoon snack

1 orange	50

Dinner

*Ham steak with orange sauce	180
2oz (55g) brown rice	66
4oz (115g) sweetcorn	86
4oz (115g) courgettes	11

Dessert

*Cranberry sorbet	50

TOTAL CALORIES	1,003

FACTS

● Table sugar (sucrose) is a carbohydrate made up of two other 'sugars', glucose, and fructose (fruit sugar), joined together in equal amounts.

● All sugars provide 4 calories per gram, less than half the amount of fat — so you could provide all your daily calorie needs with a pound (just over half a kilo) of sugar a day! But you would lack all the vitamins, minerals, and protein needed for a healthy diet.

Daily chart

Today's weight _____

Symptoms _____

_____

_____

_____

_____

WEEK 4 — DAY 2

Breakfast	Calories
2 scrambled eggs	160
2 grilled tomatoes	16
2 rice-cakes or	
1 slice of slimmer's bread	56

Mid-morning snack

4oz (115g) raw carrot	26
1 apple	50

Lunch

1 chicken drumstick	
(4oz/115g)	84
*Green salad	32
Jacket potato	96
1 teaspoon (5ml) low-fat	
spread	25
1 tablespoon (15ml) low-calorie dressing	25

Mid-afternoon snack

1 rice-cake with	
1 teaspoon low-calorie jam	38

Dinner

*Haddock parcels	180
4oz (115g) marrow	8
4oz (115g) carrots	21
4oz (115g) potatoes	90

Dessert

Fruit salad	100
TOTAL CALORIES	**1,007**

FACTS

● On average we each eat approximately 80lb (36kg) of sucrose per year in the UK.

● The highest sugar consumers are male adolescents; females consume less, and consumption decreases with age. On average, 18 per cent of our daily calories come from sugar. In children it can be as high as 50 per cent.

Daily chart

Today's weight _____

Symptoms _____

_____

_____

_____

_____

_____

WEEK 4 — DAY 3

Breakfast	Calories
1oz (30g) Rice Krispies	105
1 medium banana	80
3floz (85ml) skimmed milk	28

Mid-morning snack

2oz (55g) raw carrot	13
6oz (170g) sticks of celery	12

Lunch

*Orange and carrot soup	55
Jacket potato	96
1 teaspoon (5ml) low-fat spread	25
*Bean salad	110

Mid-afternoon snack

1 apple	50

Dinner

*Liver with orange	250
4oz (115g) cauliflower	10
4oz (115g) French beans	8
2oz (55g) brown rice	66

Dessert

*Peach sundae	95

TOTAL CALORIES	1,003

FACTS

● Honey contains some sucrose as well as glucose and fructose; 1 teaspoon of honey has the same amount of calories as one teaspoon of sucrose.

● There are no major differences in the nutritional qualities between white and brown sugar or, for that matter, honey. Fructose (fruit sugar) tastes one-and-a-half times sweeter than the equivalent weight of sucrose or glucose. Hence honey tastes sweeter, weight for weight, than plain sucrose.

Daily chart

Today's weight _____

Symptoms _____

_____

_____

_____

_____

_____

WEEK 4 — DAY 4

Breakfast	Calories
1 boiled egg	80
2 rice-cakes or	
1 piece of slimmer's	
bread	56
1 teaspoon low-calorie	
jam	10

Mid-morning snack

3½oz (100g) Shape yogurt	40
½ grated apple	25

Lunch

5oz (140g) grilled plaice	
with lemon	131
4oz (115g) potatoes	90
4oz (115g) peas	59
4oz (115g) carrots	21

Mid-afternoon snack

4oz (115g) raw carrots	26
3oz (85g) stick of celery	6

Dinner

*Prawn and vegetable	
stir-fry	225
2oz (55g) brown rice,	66
mixed with	
1oz (30g) hazelnuts	95

Dessert

*Fruit snow	70
TOTAL CALORIES	1,000

FACTS

● The world production of sugar has increased by nearly thirty times in the last hundred years. This is the largest change in any food that we now commonly consume.

● The vast majority of manufactured foods sweetened with sucrose use white refined sugar.

Daily chart

Today's weight _____

Symptoms _____

_____

_____

_____

_____

_____

WEEK 4 — DAY 5

Breakfast	Calories
1oz (30g) cornflakes	104
3floz (85ml) skimmed milk	28
1 chopped apple	50

Mid-morning snack

2 rice-cakes with 2 teaspoons low-calorie jam	76

Lunch

4oz (115g) lean ham	135
*Cole-slaw	40
*Green salad	32
1 teaspoon (5ml) low-calorie spread	25
*Brown rice salad	110

Mid-afternoon snack

1 fresh orange	50
4oz (115g) raw carrots	26

Dinner

*Spicy fish	110
4oz (115g) broccoli	20
4oz (115g) carrots	21
4oz (115g) jacket potato	96

Dessert

*Jellied grapefruit	70

TOTAL CALORIES	993

FACTS

● A high consumption of sugar is linked with obesity, heart disease, high blood pressure, appendicitis, gallstones, and many other diseases of civilization.

● Only one-third of sucrose consumption is visible, as that added to our tea and coffee or used at home. The remaining two-thirds of the sucrose we eat is in 'hidden' form, as in chocolate, confectionery, biscuits, cakes, soft drinks, and ice-cream.

Daily chart

Today's weight _____

Symptoms _____

_____

_____

_____

_____

_____

WEEK 4 — DAY 6

Breakfast	**Calories**
2 scrambled eggs	160
2 grilled tomatoes (4oz/115g)	16

Mid-morning snack

1 grated apple	50
3½oz (100g) Shape yogurt	40

Lunch

5oz (140g) tuna, canned in brine	150
2oz (55g) brown rice	66
4oz (115g) lettuce	14
4oz (115g) grated carrots	26
1 tomato (2oz/55g)	8

Mid-afternoon snack

1 rice-cake with 1 teaspoon low-calorie jam	38

Dinner

4oz (115g) grilled lean steak, fillet or rump	192
Jacket potato	96
*Beansprout salad	65

Dessert

*Baked apple	80

TOTAL CALORIES	1,001

FACTS

● In the UK, on average, men smoke seven cigarettes a day and women five cigarettes a day.

● For every £1 we spend on food, on average we spend 22p on tobacco.

● Smoking is a powerful appetite suppressant. On ceasing smoking many people gain weight, which can be 10lb (4.5kg) or even more.

Daily chart

Today's weight _____

Symptoms _____

_____

_____

_____

_____

_____

WEEK 4 — DAY 7

Breakfast	Calories
1oz (30g) Rice Krispies	105
3floz (85ml) skimmed milk	28
1 chopped orange	50

Mid-morning snack	
4oz (115g) raw carrots	26
6oz (170g) celery sticks	12

Lunch	
1 can of Weight Watchers beef and vegetable soup	70
Jacket potato, with	96
1 teaspoon (5ml) low-calorie spread	25
*Cole-slaw	40
*Courgette and cauliflower salad	27

Mid-afternoon snack	
1 apple	50

Dinner	
*Stuffed mackerel	250
4oz (115g) cauliflower	10
4oz (115g) broccoli	20
4oz (115g) sweetcorn	86

Dessert	
*Fruit salad	100

| TOTAL CALORIES | 995 |

FACTS

● In recent years, some groups have decreased their cigarette consumption. This is particularly true for men, especially those who are better educated. Many women have started smoking or increased their consumption. Smoking increases the level of cholesterol and the other fats in the blood which leads to heart disease.

● Smokers have lower levels of vitamin C. It seems they require 2–300mg per day, up to ten times the daily RDA (recommended daily amount) to bring their levels up to normal.

Daily chart

Today's weight _____

Symptoms _____

_____

_____

_____

_____

_____

WEEK-ENDING CHART
Stage I

Date

Total weight change this week	Withdrawal symptoms experienced	General degree of well-being*	Any other comments or observations
Weight at beginning of week			
Weight at end of week			
Total weight loss			

*Score degree of well-being
Very well   3   Well   2   Fair   1   Unwell   0

RECIPES

For American readers
NB: Please note the following differences between American and British cookery terms:

British	American
1 teaspoon	1¼ teaspoon
1 tablespoon	1¼ tablespoon
1 pint (20floz)	1¾ pints
8floz (225ml)	1 cup
aubergine	eggplant
bicarbonate of soda	baking soda
brewer's yeast	nutritional yeast
broad beans	fava beans
butter beans	lima beans
chick-peas	garbanzos
Chinese leaves	Bok Choy, Chinese cabbage
coriander (fresh)	cilantro
cornflour	corn starch
courgettes	zucchini
crushed (garlic, etc.)	minced
French beans	snap beans
frying pan	skillet
haricot beans	navy beans
jam	jelly
jelly	jello
liquidize	blend
mangetout	snow peas
marrow	summer squash
minced (beef)	ground
natural yogurt	plain yogurt
pancake	crepe
sieve	strain
slimmer's	dieter's
spring greens	collards
spring onion	scallion
swede	rutabaga
tomato purée	tomato paste
wholemeal	whole wheat

Cumin chicken

Serves 2   Calories per serving 145

2×4oz (115g) chicken breast fillets, cubed
3 spring onions, chopped
½ red pepper, chopped
1 teaspoon cumin seeds
1 teaspoon vegetable oil
1 teaspoon finely chopped root ginger
Cornflour
Water

1. Heat oil in saucepan, add the cumin seeds, stir until they start popping.
2. Add chicken, pepper, onions and ginger; stir for 3 minutes.
3. Add the stock, bring to the boil, simmer for 5 minutes.
4. Add cornflour (mixed into paste with water), and simmer for a further 5 minutes before serving.

Liver with orange

Serves 2   Calories per serving 250

6oz (170g) lamb's liver, thinly sliced
1 small onion (2oz/55g) thinly sliced
½ green pepper (2oz/55g) cored and diced
1×3oz (55g) rasher of lean bacon, sliced into 1-inch (2.5cm) pieces
2 oranges, separated into segments and chopped in half
4floz (115ml) orange juice
1 tablespoon (15ml) oil
1 tablespoon flour, seasoned with freshly ground black pepper

1. Gently fry the onion in the oil for about 2–5 minutes.
2. Add the pepper, bacon, and liver coated in seasoned flour and fry for a further minute.
3. Add the orange juice and simmer for 5 minutes.
4. Add the halved orange segments, heat through for 1 minute and serve.

Stuffed mackerel

Serves 2   Calories per serving 250

2 × 5oz (140g) fresh mackerel, gutted
1 apple, grated
2 tablespoons cooked brown rice
1 medium onion, finely chopped
1 orange
1 teaspoon dried rosemary *or*
    4 sprigs fresh rosemary
1 tablespoon parsley, finely chopped

1. Grate peel of orange and chop flesh into small pieces, discarding pips.
2. Mix orange, apple, parsley, onion and rice together.
3. Divide mixture into two and use to stuff mackerel loosely.
4. Place rosemary in each fish.
5. Bake in foil for about 40 minutes at 200°C/400°F/Gas Mark 6.

Chicken paprika

Serves 4   Calories per serving 220

4 × 5oz (140g) chicken joints
2 teaspoons paprika pepper
5½floz (155ml) vegetable stock
1 onion, finely chopped
Freshly ground black pepper
1 tablespoon finely chopped parsley
1–2 teaspoons cornflour mixed with a tablespoon of water

1. Sprinkle chicken with paprika.
2. Gently grill on both sides for about 5 minutes until brown.
3. Place in a casserole dish with vegetable stock, onion and freshly ground black pepper.
4. Cover and simmer for 30–40 minutes or until tender.
5. Lift out chicken, place on a warm dish and cover to keep hot.
6. Thicken liquid with cornflour. Pour over chicken and serve, decorate with a pinch of fresh parsley.

Tomato jacket

Serves 1   Calories 119

1×4oz (115g) baking potato
3 fresh tomatoes
Freshly ground black pepper
½ teaspoon mixed herbs

1. Bake potato, remove from oven and cut in half lengthways. Scoop out the inside and mash until smooth.
2. Skin and chop fresh tomatoes, add ½ teaspoon of mixed herbs and a little black pepper.
3. Mix tomato and potato together and spoon back into the potato jacket.
4. Place under grill until top is lightly browned.

Vegetable curry

Serves 2   Calories per serving 185

6oz (170g) boiled butter beans
3oz (85g) cauliflower, broken into florets
3oz (85g) turnip, cut into 1-inch (2.5cm) cubes
3oz (85g) parsnip, cut into 1-inch (2.5cm) cubes
3oz (85g) courgettes, thickly sliced
1 small onion, chopped
½ small chilli, seeded and finely chopped
2 tablespoons tomato purée
1½ pints (30floz/850ml) vegetable stock
¼ teaspoon turmeric
¼ teaspoon coriander
¼ teaspoon cumin seeds
1 teaspoon finely chopped ginger
1 garlic clove, crushed
2 teaspoons vegetable oil

1. Heat oil in a saucepan. Add garlic, spices and chilli, and stir over a moderate heat for 2 minutes.
2. Add all remaining ingredients, mix well and bring to the boil.
3. Cover and simmer for 15 minutes, then for a further 10 minutes without lid.
4. Serve with brown rice and small salad.

Liver kebabs

Serves 4   Calories per serving 225

1lb (455g) lamb's liver, cut into bite-size pieces
8 small onions, peeled and blanched
8 small tomatoes
8 pineapple cubes
1 tablespoon (15ml) of vegetable oil
Freshly ground black pepper

1. Thread 8 skewers with liver, onion, tomato, and pineapple.
2. Brush with oil, season with pepper.
3. Cook under hot grill for about 8 minutes.
4. Serve with brown rice and/or salad.

Haddock parcels

Serves 4   Calories per serving 180

4×5oz (140g) haddock cutlets
6oz (170g) courgettes, thinly sliced
8oz (225g) tomatoes, peeled and thinly sliced
8oz (225g) celery, sliced
1 red and 1 green pepper, seeded and sliced
4oz (115g) of canned sweetcorn
2 tablespoons (30ml) lemon juice
2 tablespoons (30ml) vegetable stock or water
1 tablespoon (15ml) freshly chopped parsley
Freshly ground black pepper

1. Place each fish on a piece of foil.
2. Simmer the vegetables in the lemon juice and stock for 10 minutes.
3. Separate vegetables into four portions and pile on top of fish.
4. Add black pepper and sprinkle with fresh parsley.
5. Wrap up fish in the foil and bake in the oven at 180°C/350°F/Gas Mark 4 for about 30 minutes.
6. Serve with vegetables or rice.

Orange and carrot soup

Serves 2   Calories per serving 55

This can be used as a sauce for grilled or roast meats, or cold as a salad dressing.

10oz (285g) carrots, chopped
1 medium leek, thinly sliced
12floz (360ml) vegetable stock
Pinch of thyme
3–4floz (85–115ml) orange juice
Freshly ground black pepper

1. Place the carrots, leek, vegetable stock and thyme into a saucepan, bring to the boil and simmer for 30 minutes.
2. Purée the mixture in a blender or food processor.
3. Return to the saucepan and add the orange juice, season with pepper.

Lamb and aubergine bake

Serves 2   Calories per serving 260

9oz (255g) aubergine
2 teaspoons vegetable oil
1 clove garlic, finely chopped
1 small onion, chopped
1 tablespoon canned sweetcorn
½oz (15g) cooked brown rice
7oz (200g) minced lamb
1 tablespoon tomato purée

1. Cut aubergine in half lengthways. Lightly score inside each half with a sharp knife. Sprinkle with salt and leave for 20–30 minutes, then rinse thoroughly in cold water.
2. Remove and chop white flesh, reserving the hollow halves.
3. Heat oil, and gently fry onion and garlic for 2–3 minutes. Add the white aubergine flesh and stir round for 2 more minutes.
4. Add the rice, sweetcorn, lamb, and tomato purée to the pan, season with pepper, and stir 2–3 minutes to brown the meat.
5. Spoon this mixture into the aubergine halves, cover and bake 190°C/375°F/Gas Mark 5 for 20–25 minutes.
6. Remove and serve immediately.

Prawn and vegetable stir-fry

Serves 4   Calories per serving 225

8oz (225g) peeled prawns
4oz (115g) onions, chopped
4oz (115g) broccoli, divided into
  florets
4oz (115g) carrots, cut into small
  matchstick size pieces
4oz (115g) leek, thinly sliced
2oz (55g) courgettes, thinly sliced
4oz (115g) Chinese leaves, roughly
  chopped
1 tablespoon (15ml) lemon juice
3 tablespoons (45ml) vegetable oil
1 tablespoon grated ginger
1 apple, cored and diced

1. Heat oil in a wok or large frying
   pan, add the broccoli, carrots and
   leeks and cook for 3 minutes.
2. Add the prawns, courgettes,
   Chinese leaves, apple, ginger,
   onions and lemon juice.
3. Fry for a further 2 minutes.
4. Serve immediately.

Kidney casserole

Serves 2   Calories per serving 270

12oz (340g) lamb's kidney
1½oz (45g) flour, seasoned with
  black pepper
1 tablespoon oil
1 small onion, chopped
1 green pepper, seeded and cut into
  strips
½ pint (285ml) vegetable stock
2 teaspoons English mustard

1. Remove kidney skins and cut
   kidneys in half.
2. Turn the kidney halves in flour.
3. Heat oil in a saucepan, add
   onion, and fry for 2 minutes.
4. Add kidney and pepper and stir
   until kidneys are lightly
   browned.
5. Stir in remaining flour, stock and
   mustard.
6. Bring to the boil, cover, reduce
   heat and simmer gently for 15
   minutes, stirring occasionally.

Salmon and scrambled eggs

Serves 2   Calories per serving 180

3 eggs
1 tablespoon skimmed milk
2 teaspoons chopped dill
Freshly ground black pepper
3oz (85g) tinned salmon

1. Whisk eggs and milk with dill and freshly ground pepper.
2. Cook gently in a non-stick pan, stirring constantly, for 4–5 minutes until firm.
3. Mix in the salmon and serve.

Pork with pineapple sauce

Serves 2   Calories per serving 220

2 × 4oz (115g) pork chops (remove any fat)
1 red and 1 green pepper, seeded and chopped
4oz (115g) canned pineapple, chopped
2–3 teaspoons cornflour
½ pint (285ml) pineapple juice

1. Place the chops under grill for 5 minutes to brown slightly.
2. Place the pork chops, pineapple and chopped peppers into a casserole dish.
3. Add the pineapple juice.
4. Cover and cook in oven for 1¼ hours at 220°C/420°F/Gas Mark 5.
5. When cooked, mix the cornflour with a little water and use to thicken sauce.

Haddock Florentine

Serves 2   Calories per serving 170

2 × 5oz (140g) haddock portions
8oz (225g) frozen spinach, defrosted and drained
2 tablespoons (30ml) of lemon juice
Slices of lemon

1. Place each haddock portion onto a piece of aluminium foil.
2. Cover each portion with half the spinach and 1 tablespoon of lemon juice and wrap in the foil.
3. Bake for 20–30 minutes at 220°C/420°F/Gas Mark 5.
4. Remove foil and serve with a slice of lemon to garnish.

Ham steaks with orange sauce

Serves 2   Calories per serving 180

2×4oz (115g) ham steaks
4floz (115ml) orange juice
1 orange, peeled and chopped
1 teaspoon (5ml) cornflour
4 tablespoons (60ml) water
Lemon juice to taste

1. Pour the orange juice into a pan. Add the chopped orange.
2. Blend the cornflour to a paste with the water. Stir into the orange juice and flesh mixture. Bring to the boil, stirring continuously.
3. Reduce the heat and simmer for 2 minutes. Add the lemon juice.
4. While the sauce is simmering, grill the ham steaks for 7–8 minutes, turning once.
5. Pour the orange sauce over the ham steaks.
6. Serve garnished with a sprig of parsley and twist of orange.

Spicy fish

Serves 4   Calories per serving 110

1lb (455g) cod fillet, skinned and cut into 4 equal pieces
3 large tomatoes, skinned and sliced
½ red pepper, seeded and chopped
½ green pepper, seeded and chopped
1 clove of garlic, crushed
1 teaspoon freshly chopped parsley
1 teaspoon freshly chopped basil
1 onion, thinly sliced
1 courgette, thinly sliced
Pinch of grated ginger
3 tablespoons (45ml) lemon juice
½ pint (285ml) vegetable water or water
Freshly ground black pepper

1. Place half the tomato slices in a casserole dish and cover with garlic, peppers, courgettes, onion and basil.
2. Season with pepper and ginger and sprinkle with half the parsley.
3. Arrange the cod on top, with the other half of the parsley, and cover with the remaining tomatoes.
4. Pour on the lemon juice and stock.
5. Cover and cook in the oven (180°C/350°F/Gas Mark 4) for about 40 minutes.
6. Serve immediately.

Beansprout salad

Side salad serves 4
Calories per serving 65

6oz (170g) beansprouts
4oz (115g) red pepper
4oz (115g) canned sweetcorn
  (drained)
2 apples, shredded/grated
4 spring onions

Bean and sweetcorn salad

Side salad serves 4
Calories per serving 25

8oz (225g) French beans, cooked,
  cooled and cut into 1-inch (2.5cm)
  lengths
4oz (115g) can of sweetcorn
2 small spring onions, sliced
Sesame seeds to garnish

Green salad

Serves 1   Calories 32

2oz (55g) lettuce
8 slices thinly-cut cucumber
½ green pepper (3oz/85g)
2oz (55g) watercress

Brown rice salad

Serves 2   Calories per serving 110

4oz (115g) brown rice
3oz (85g) sweetcorn (canned)
½ red pepper (3oz/85g)
½ green pepper (3oz/85g)

Potato salad

Serves 2   Calories per serving 125

8oz (225g) boiled potatoes, chopped
  into bite-size pieces
2 spring onions, chopped
2 tablespoons low-calorie dressing
2 teaspoons snipped fresh chives

Cauliflower and carrot salad

Serves 2   Calories per serving 30

4oz (115g) raw carrot, cut into small
  sticks
4oz (115g) raw cauliflower, cut into
  small sprigs
4oz (115g) chopped cucumber
½ level teaspoon mixed herbs

Vegetable salad

Side salad serves 4
Calories per serving 50

4oz (115g) frozen peas
3oz (85g) French beans
4oz (115g) canned sweetcorn
¼ red pepper
1 tablespoon freshly chopped
  parsley

Bean salad

Side salad serves 4   Calories per serving 110

4oz (115g) broad beans
4oz (115g) red kidney beans (canned)
4oz (115g) haricot beans (soaked overnight)
4oz (115g) chick-peas (soaked overnight)
2 tablespoons (30ml) finely chopped parsley
1 medium onion, finely chopped
½ teaspoon (2.5ml) cumin seeds, ground
2 tablespoons (30ml) cold-pressed olive or vegetable oil
1 bay leaf
2 sprigs of thyme
1 clove garlic, crushed (optional)

1. Drain the haricot beans and chick-peas, and cover with water in a saucepan. Boil for 10 minutes, then add the bay leaf and sprigs of thyme, and simmer for 1 to 1½ hours. Drain and leave to cool.
2. Mix the garlic with the oil and kidney and broad beans. Pour over remaining beans.
3. Add the parsley, cumin seeds and onion.

Beetroot cabbage salad

Serves 4   Calories per serving 47

6oz (170g) raw beetroot, grated
6oz (170g) firm white cabbage, shredded
6oz (170g) red cabbage, grated
6oz (170g) carrots, grated
1 small onion, finely chopped
½ red pepper, cored, seeded and chopped
1oz (30g) sunflower seeds

1. Mix all ingredients, leaving the beetroot until just before serving.

Root salad

Side salad serves 4   Calories per serving 31

4oz (115g) celeriac root
6oz (170g) carrots
4oz (115g) parsnip
3oz (85g) beetroot

1. Chop or grate celeriac, carrots, and parsnips and mix together.
2. Chop beetroot and sprinkle on top of salad.

Stuffed pepper

Serves 1   Calories per serving 163

1 medium green pepper
2oz (55g) cooked brown rice
½ apple, chopped
2oz (55g) canned sweetcorn
2oz (55g) carrot, shredded

1. Halve the pepper lengthways, scoop out seeds and steam for 10 minutes.
2. Mix other ingredients together and use to stuff pepper.
3. Place in oven-proof dish, cover and cook for 15 minutes at 200°C/400°F/Gas Mark 6.

Tomato sauce

Serves 4   Calories per serving 35

4oz (115g) onion, finely chopped
1 clove garlic, crushed
14oz (385g) fresh ripe tomatoes, chopped and skin removed, *or*
  1 tin (14oz/385g) plum tomatoes, drained and chopped
2 teaspoons olive oil
½ teaspoon mixed herbs or basil
Freshly ground black pepper to taste

1. Heat the oil, add onion and garlic, cover, and cook gently for 5 minutes until the onion is soft.
2. Add the tomatoes and herbs. Cover and cook for 15 minutes.
3. Season with fresh black pepper.
4. Cool if serving sauce as salad dressing.

Cole-slaw

Serves 4   Calories per serving 40

1lb (455g) white cabbage, shredded
4oz (115g) carrots, grated
1 onion, sliced
2 tablespoons slimmer's
   mayonnaise or dressing or natural
   slimmer's yogurt
1 tablespoon finely choped fresh
   parsley to garnish

Tomato and celery salad

Side salad serves 4
Calories per serving 20

8oz (225g) tomatoes, cut into 8
   pieces
4oz (115g) celery, chopped
4oz (115g) green pepper
4oz (115g) lettuce, shredded
1 tablespoon freshly chopped
   parsley to garnish

Courgette and cauliflower salad

Side salad serves 4
Calories per serving 27

3oz (85g) courgettes, thinly sliced
8oz (225g) cauliflower, cut into
   small florets
4oz (115g) red pepper, cored and
   chopped
1 apple, cored and chopped
1 teaspoon freshly chopped fennel
   to garnish

Ginger and carrot salad

Side salad serves 4
Calories per serving 36

6oz (170g) carrots, grated
2 medium apples, grated
1 teaspoon ground ginger
1 stick of celery, chopped

Fruity cabbage salad

Side salad serves 4
Calories per serving 75

1lb (455g) white cabbage, shredded
4oz (115g) green pepper, chopped
5 radishes, sliced
1 red and 1 green apple, chopped
1 medium orange, broken into
   segments and halved
4oz (115g) chopped melon

Summer salad

Serves 4   Calories per serving 45

4oz (115g) courgettes
3oz (85g) carrots
3oz (85g) baby turnips
2oz (55g) spinach leaves
8oz (225g) broad beans

Melon and pilchard salad

Serves 1   Calories 241

4oz (115g) pilchards
4oz (115g) lettuce
*Fruity cabbage salad

Fruit salad

Serves 4   Calories per serving 100

1 dessert apple, peeled and sliced
1 banana, peeled and sliced
4 tablespoons (60ml) lemon juice
1 orange, peeled and segmented
1 grapefruit, peeled and segmented
4oz (115g) seedless grapes
2 kiwi fruits, peeled and sliced
2 tablespoons (30ml) orange juice
4 sprigs of mint

1. Toss the apple and banana in the lemon juice. This will prevent discolouration.
2. Combine all fruits in a serving bowl, serve chilled and decorate with a sprig of mint.

Gooseberry jelly

Serves 6   Calories per serving 70

1lb (455g) gooseberries, topped and tailed
½ pint (285ml) pure apple juice
¼ pint (140ml) water
4 teaspoons powdered gelatine
Concentrated apple juice to sweeten
Gooseberries to decorate

1. Very sparingly, oil a 1½-pint (30floz/850ml) jelly mould.
2. Simmer the gooseberries and water until soft.
3. Blend the fruit in the liquidizer.
4. Mix this purée with the apple juice, and a little extra concentrated apple juice to sweeten according to taste.
5. Mix the gelatine with two tablespoons of water in a small heat-proof bowl, place the bowl in hot water and stir until dissolved.
6. Add the gooseberry mixture to the gelatine mixture and mix thoroughly.
7. Pour into the prepared jelly mould and chill for 2–3 hours until set.
8. Turn the jelly carefully out onto a serving plate and decorate with gooseberries.

Cranberry sorbet

Serves 4   Calories per serving 50

8oz (225g) fresh cranberries
½ pint (285ml) water
½ pint (285ml) unsweetened orange juice
2 egg whites
Artificial sweetener to taste if necessary

1. Place the orange juice and cranberries in a saucepan together with the water. Bring to the boil. Cover saucepan and simmer gently for 2–3 minutes.
2. Strain the cranberries, keeping the cranberry juice in a separate bowl.
3. Blend the soft cranberries in a liquidizer and add the juices.
4. Allow to cool and add the sweetener, if necessary.
5. Put the cranberry mixture into a shallow dish and place in the freezer until semi-frozen.
6. Whisk the egg whites until stiff.
7. Remove the cranberry mixture from the freezer and break up the ice crystals that have formed.
8. Tip the semi-frozen sorbet into a bowl and fold in the whisked egg white.
9. Return the mixture to the container and freeze until firm.
10. When you are ready to serve, scoop the Cranberry sorbet into decorative glasses.

Peach sundae

Serves 2　Calories per serving 95

2 peaches
5oz (140g) raspberries
2½ teaspoons sugar
1 teaspoon arrowroot
2 teaspoons shredded, or toasted,
　desiccated coconut

1. Skin the peaches by blanching them. (Pour boiling water over them, leave to cool briefly, and then place in cold water. The skins will then peel off easily.)
2. Halve the peaches and remove the stones.
3. Sieve the raspberries, making a purée.
4. Take a little of the raspberry purée and mix with the arrowroot into a paste.
5. Stir the arrowroot paste into the raspberry purée, and add sugar.
6. Place the mixture in a saucepan and boil for 1 minute, stirring constantly.
7. When the mixture has cooled, pour the sauce over the peaches and sprinkle with the coconut.

Baked apple

Serves 1　Calories 80

1 cooking apple
1 dessertspoon of concentrated
　apple juice
1 cup of water
1 pinch of cinnamon

1. Wash and core the apple, and score around the centre of the apple in a circle just breaking the skin.
2. Place the apple in an oven-proof dish.
3. Mix the concentrated apple juice with the water and the cinnamon.
4. Pour the water into the dish, and pour the apple juice over the apple.
5. Bake in a moderate oven 180°C/ 350°F/Gas Mark 4 for approximately 50–60 minutes.

Fruit snow

Serves 2   Calories per serving 70

7oz (200g) dessert apples, peeled,
  cored and thinly sliced
Grated orange rind
2 tablespoons (30ml) water
1 large egg white, beaten until stiff
Orange slices for garnish

1. Place apple, water and orange rind in a saucepan. Cover and cook gently, stirring occasionally until apples are soft.
2. Rub the apples through a sieve and let them cool.
3. Fold in the egg white and chill before serving. Serve with a slice of orange to decorate.

Rhubarb and ginger mousse

Serves 4   Calories per serving 50

1lb (455g) rhubarb
Juice and grated rind of half an
  orange
3 tablespoons clear honey
2 egg whites
2 tablespoons (30ml) water
¼ teaspoon ground ginger
2 teaspoons powdered gelatine

1. Trim the rhubarb and chop into 1-inch (2.5cm) pieces.
2. Put the rhubarb into a pan with the honey, orange juice, rind and the ginger, and simmer gently until the fruit is soft.
3. Dissolve the gelatine in 2 tablespoons of water, placing the bowl in hot water. Stir until the gelatine is dissolved.
4. Add the gelatine mixture to the fruit and beat until smooth.
5. Cool the rhubarb mixture until it is half-set.
6. Whisk the egg whites until stiff and fold them lightly into the half-set rhubarb mixture.
7. Spoon into decorative glasses and chill until set.

Jellied grapefruit

Serves 4   Calories per serving 70

2 large pink grapefruits, halved
½ pint (285ml) unsweetened
  pineapple juice
¼ pint (140ml) unsweetened
  grapefruit juice
3 teaspoons gelatine

1. Scoop out the grapefruit
   segments from the grapefruit.
   Remove any pith from the
   segments and from the grapefruit
   shells.
2. Place the four grapefruit shells
   on a dish and divide the
   grapefruit segments evenly
   among them.
3. Mix together the fruit juices.
   Take two tablespoons of mixed
   juices and add to the gelatine.
   Place the bowl in hot water, and
   stir until the gelatine has
   dissolved.
4. Mix the gelatine solution with
   the remaining fruit juice
   mixture. Pour equal amounts
   into each grapefruit shell.
5. Place the shells in the fridge to
   set.

PACKED LUNCHES

If you are working full-time, or even
part-time, you may need to take food
with you to work. Some work
canteens do serve salads or jacket
potatoes, which will be useful when
you reach Stage III of the diet, but
initially it is important that the
weight and calorie content of your
diet is exact or as near as possible. It
is, therefore, better if you prepare your
own lunches initially, rather than rely
on canteens.

Planning is all-important. When
preparing your evening meal, give a
thought to tomorrow's lunch. You can
boil some brown rice and leave to cool
for tomorrow. Make an extra portion
of salad if you are eating salad that
evening, and leave it in the fridge to be
collected as you leave for work in the
morning.

In Stage I you will need to avoid all
the wheat, dairy, yeast and other
foods in your packed lunches. In Stage
II you can use the foods that you are
introducing for that week. Some
examples are listed below to help you.
Where an asterisk (*) is marked you
will find the dish in the Recipe
section.

	Calories		**Calories**
*Brown rice salad, with 5oz (140g) tin sardines (in tomato sauce), 1 apple	410	4oz (115g) peeled prawns, *Courgette and cauliflower salad, 2oz (55g) brown rice	212
4oz (115g) tinned tuna (in brine), with *Green salad and *Potato salad	218	One hard-boiled egg, *Fruity cabbage salad, *Potato salad	270
4oz (115g) cold chicken breast or drumstick (without skin), 4oz (115g) grated carrot, 1 tomato cut into 8, 3oz (85g) of sliced celery, 4oz (115g) shredded white cabbage, 1 tablespoon (15ml) low-calorie dressing	146	*Bean salad, 1 chopped apple, 4oz (115g) lettuce	226
4oz (115g) cold lean ham, *Beansprout salad and 2oz (55g) brown rice	266	Three rice-cakes with sardines (in tomato sauce), *or* 4oz (115g) sardines mixed with 1 tablespoon (15ml) low-calorie dressing spread onto three crispbreads with two slices of tomato on each	300
4oz (115g) cold lean beef, *Tomato and celery salad, 2oz (55g) *Potato salad	318	4oz (115g) cold pork with *Green salad, 2 tomatoes	287
		*Stuffed pepper	163
		*Melon and pilchard salad	241
		4oz (115g) salmon with *Green salad and *Potato salad	332

20
Stage II —
the challenge begins

First of all, take a pat on the back for successfully completing the first four weeks of the diet. You should be feeling slimmer and healthier than when you began. The next four weeks require the most skill and perseverance. You will be experimenting to identify any foods that may be causing you health problems and weight gain.

Stage II is broken down into four sections of one week each. There is a specific diet to follow for each of the four weeks. Each week, you will be concentrating on eating a specific group of foods and carefully noting any reactions or changes in your physical or mental well-being that may occur.

For each day there is a diet sheet, more interesting key facts, and a weight and symptom chart for you to complete as you did for Stage I. It is vital that you keep this chart up to date: you will undoubtedly need to refer back at some point during the next few weeks, so the records are nothing short of vital!

At the end of each of the following four weeks there is a recipe section which you might like to try if you have the time and the inclination. Unless you absolutely hate cooking it is advisable to experiment with some of the recipes in order to keep the diet interesting. It really is not necessary to get bored with eating the same foods during the next four weeks.

Desserts are suggested especially for each of the four weeks of Stage II, as there are more specific requirements for these weeks. Desserts can be substituted by a portion of fresh fruit, or fresh fruit salad, but if possible in Stage II try to prepare the suggested desserts from the recipes provided.

Follow the suggested menus each day, introducing new foods as directed and keeping within the framework of 1,000 calories per day. If you experience the return of any symptoms, or any new symptoms, during this week, mark them down on your daily chart, and go back to the diet in Stage I for the remainder of that week only.

SUSPECT FOODS

Any foods that you suspect are

causing problems during the course of Stage II must immediately be struck out of your diet. This is very important. Failure to eliminate a suspect food will undoubtedly cause confusion and cloud the whole picture. It's far better to be safe than sorry! If you even mildly suspect a particular food may be causing a problem, set that food aside, for now at least. It will be possible for you to retest potentially suspect foods later on, *but not during Stage II*.

We cannot emphasize enough how important it is to set aside from your diet foods you suspect or know cause you problems.

YOUR QUESTIONS ANSWERED

How do I tell if I'm reacting to a food?

Sensitivities to foods manifest themselves in many different ways. For example, a reaction to a particular food *may occur within a few minutes of eating a food, or after a day or two.* It is for this reason that we allow a whole week to try eating each group of foods. It gives you plenty of time to be certain about whether the food suits you or not without confusing the issue.

What sort of reaction can I expect?

The types of reaction to food are also very varied. Any of the following signs

or symptoms may cause you to be suspicious:

water retention	asthma
abdominal bloating	migraine headache
abdominal wind	insomnia
abdominal pain	anxiety or irritability
diarrhoea, constipation	eczema
puffy eyelids	rhinitis (sneezing or a runny nose)
swollen fingers or ankles	

What happens if I get a mild reaction?

If you get only a mild reaction to a particular food, watch it carefully until it either disappears or increases into a full-blown reaction.

What happens if I don't usually eat or drink the foods in one of the sections of Stage II?

If you genuinely don't eat *any* of the foods that we suggest you test in one of the weeks of Stage II, there will be no need for you to follow the instructions for that week However, if you consume some of the foods or drinks then it is advisable to include that week. For example, on Week 3 of Stage II, you are asked to concentrate on consuming foods containing yeast or alcohol. If you don't drink alcohol but do usually eat bread, marmite, and vinegar, you should undertake this week, concentrating on those foods.

IMPORTANT NOTE

During Stage II you may well find that you will need to give up one or both of your snacks each day in order to make way for the higher calorie foods that you will be adding to your diet. Plan your menus in advance at the beginning of each of the next four weeks. So, for example, if you want to eat more foods containing dairy produce in Week 2, or more chocolate-containing foods in Week 4, you will need to compensate by dropping your mid-morning and possibly your mid-afternoon snack.

21
Week I — wheat and other grains

During the first week of Stage II you are going to introduce grains back into your diet. We will concentrate mainly on foods containing wheat, because these seem to be the culprits more commonly than other grains — perhaps because they are more commonly consumed. However, if your usual diet incorporated oats, barley or rye or if you would like to experiment, you can include foods containing these this week.

JULIE ASPINALL

For a year after the birth of her third child Julie was two stones (28lb/12.5kg) overweight.

'I tried 1,000 calories per day diets. In fact, my doctor even put me on a diet. I did manage to lose half a stone [7lb/3kg], but I was so hungry all the time that I could not keep the diet up for longer than a month. I only felt well for one out of every four weeks. I had abdominal wind and suffered with thrush on and off.

'When I began the WNAS diet I was asked to cut out bread, biscuits and cakes as well as cutting down on dairy products and sugar, I found that I was sensitive to wheat. I was given exercise recommendations to follow as well.

'I lost one-and-a-half stones in three months on the WNAS programme. I'm now down to the weight my doctor said I should be. Whereas on other diets I had felt hungry and unwell, on the WNAS diet I didn't feel hungry at all and I felt very well. All my abdominal bloating symptoms disappeared as well as the indigestion and heartburn that I always used to suffer with.

'Apart from being stably slimmer in that I have managed to maintain the weight loss this time, I feel a great deal better in myself. I can cope with things in a better manner and am able to take on far more. My husband says I am calmer and more relaxed and that I have had a much more positive outlook on life.'

WEEK 1 — DAY 1

Breakfast	Calories
2 Weetabix (1oz/30g)	96
3floz (85ml) skimmed milk	28
1 chopped apple	50

Mid-morning snack

1 slice of wholemeal toast	70
1 teaspoon low-calorie spread	25
2 teaspoons low-calorie jam	20

Lunch

1oz (30g) sweetcorn	21
1 scrambled egg (size 3)	80
1 slice of wholemeal toast	70

Mid-afternoon snack

4oz (115g) raw carrots	26

Dinner

*Fish crumble	385
4oz (115g) courgettes	11
4oz (115g) carrots	21

Dessert

*Lemon fruit roll	96

TOTAL CALORIES	999

FACTS

● The term 'fibre' refers to the parts of our food that are indigestible by the human digestive tract and go to form the majority of waste from the gut.

● Fibre is almost entirely of plant origin. Small amounts may come from shellfish. In the main, most of the fibre in plants is found in their supporting structures and thus is in the walls of cells and the outer parts of the plant, e.g. stems or skins, rather than the leaves or inner part.

Daily chart

Today's weight _____

Symptoms _____

_____

_____

_____

_____

WEEK 1 — DAY 2

Breakfast	**Calories**
½oz (15g) porridge (raw weight) made with water	44
½ apple, chopped	25

Mid-morning snack

1 slice of wholemeal toast	70
1 teaspoon (5ml) low-calorie jam	10
1 teaspoon low-calorie spread	25

Lunch

2oz (55g) lean ham, in a salad sandwich	67
2 slices of wholemeal bread	140
½oz (15g) lettuce	1
1 sliced tomato (2oz/55g)	8
1 teaspoon low-calorie spread	25

Mid-afternoon snack

1 piece of fresh fruit	50

Dinner

*Chicken and sweetcorn lasagne	350
*Green salad	32

Dessert

*Apple Charlotte	155
TOTAL CALORIES	1,002

FACTS

● The slower the passage of food fibre and food residues through the colon, the greater the breakdown of the fibre and release of energy. Women, who have slower moving bowels than men, could derive a few calories less than 50 a day.

● As fibre-rich waste products are broken down in the large bowel, a number of products are formed apart from the release of calories. Gases, especially, are formed from certain types of fibre, leading to flatulence (wind). The fibre of beans and lentils are easily turned into some foul-smelling wind by this process.

Daily chart

Today's weight _____

Symptoms _____

_____

_____

_____

_____

_____

WEEK 1 — DAY 3

Breakfast	Calories
2 slices of wholemeal toast	140
1 grilled tomato (2oz/55g)	8
1 poached egg (size 3)	80

Mid-morning snack

6oz (170g) sticks of celery	12

Lunch

8oz (225g) Weight Watchers baked beans	122
1 piece of wholemeal toast	70

Mid-afternoon snack

2oz (55g) raw carrot	13

Dinner

*Lentil rissoles	290
*Ginger and carrot salad	36
4oz (115g) lettuce	14
4oz (115g) new potatoes	90

Dessert

*Sponge cake	140
TOTAL CALORIES	**1,015**

FACTS

● Different types of fibre may help to protect you against different types of disease. Fibre from cereals such as wheat bran or wholemeal bread may be good for constipation, but the fibre from fruit and vegetables is associated with a lower risk of appendictis and coronary heart disease.

● On average, fruits contain 1–3g of fibre per 100g (3½oz) and green vegetables 2–4g. Peas have 7g, cooked beans 10g, baked beans 7g, dried fruit 10g, dried figs 17g, nuts 5–10g, wholemeal bread 9g, and finally brown and white rice less than 1g.

Daily chart

Today's weight _____

Symptoms _____

_____

_____

_____

_____

_____

WEEK 1 — DAY 4

Breakfast	Calories
2oz (55g) Jordan's Special Muesli	95
3floz (85ml) skimmed milk	28
½ grated apple	25

Mid-morning snack

1 slice of wholemeal toast	70
1 teaspoon (5ml) low-calorie jam	10
1 teaspoon low-calorie spread	25

Lunch

*Pizza toast	280
*Root salad	31

Mid-afternoon snack

2oz (55g) raw carrot	13

Dinner

*Wholewheat spaghetti with ham and spinach sauce	275
*Tomato and celery salad	20
1 tablespoon (15ml) low-calorie dressing	25

Dessert

*Carrot and date cake	115
TOTAL CALORIES	1,012

FACTS

● The greatest consumers of fruit and vegetables are the Italians, French, and Swiss.

● The greatest consumers of beans and pulses are the Japanese.

● The greatest consumers of root vegetables are the French, Belgians, and Irish.

● The greatest consumers of wheat fibre are the Slavs (from Yugoslavia) and the Greeks.

● The greatest consumers of corn are the Mexicans.

● The greatest consumers of rice are the Japanese, Chinese and Singaporeans, and the Scandinavians are the largest consumers of rye.

Daily chart

Today's weight _____

Symptoms _____

_____

_____

_____

_____

_____

WEEK 1 — DAY 5

Breakfast	Calories
1oz (30g) branflakes	85
3floz (85ml) skimmed milk	28
½ apple, grated	25

Mid-morning snack

4oz (115g) raw carrots	26

Lunch

2oz (55g) chicken in a sandwich	245
*Ginger and carrot salad	36

Mid-afternoon snack

1 fresh orange	50

Dinner

*Beef and spinach pasta	310
*Green salad	32
1 tablespoon (15ml) low-calorie dressing	25

Dessert

*Apple scone	170

TOTAL CALORIES	1,007

FACTS

● To obtain your recommended daily intake of fibre, approx. 30g, you would need to consume: 1,000 calories worth of brown bread, 3,000 calories of white bread, 1,400 calories of corn/maize, 1,400 calories of brown or white rice, 1,100 calories of root vegetables, 600 calories of pulses, 2,000 calories of peanuts, 300 calories of green vegetables, or 600 calories of fruit.

● The richest source of fibre and lowest source of calories are therefore green vegetables, beans and fruit.

Daily chart

Today's weight _____

Symptoms _____

_____

_____

_____

_____

_____

WEEK 1 — DAY 6

Breakfast	**Calories**
1 scrambled egg (size 3)	80
1 slice of wholemeal toast	70

Mid-morning snack

1 slice of wholemeal toast with 1 teaspoon low-calorie jam	80

Lunch

2oz (55g) prawns with tomato and lettuce in a wholemeal roll	215

Mid-afternoon snack

½ grated apple	25
3oz (85g) stick celery	6

Dinner

*Turkey in wholemeal breadcrumbs	254
4oz (115g) broccoli	20
4oz (115g) courgettes	11
4oz (115g) new potatoes	90

Dessert

*Pancakes (wholemeal) with lemon and sugar	150
TOTAL CALORIES	**1,001**

FACTS

- Iron availability from fibre-rich vegetarian foods can be quite poor and worsened by wheat bran if taken in large amounts. This effect is reduced if extra vitamin C (e.g. one or two pieces of fruit) is eaten at the same time.

- Fibre-rich diets may help with weight loss by: reducing the amount of calories in the same volume of food; increasing the amount of chewing and so slowing the rate of intake; increasing the feeling of satisfaction; helping to balance the body's glucose and hormonal metabolisms; and being more nutritious.

Daily chart

Today's weight _____

Symptoms _____

_____

_____

_____

_____

_____

WEEK 1 — DAY 7

Breakfast	Calories
2oz (55g) Jordan's Special Muesli	95
3floz (85ml) skimmed milk	28
½ chopped apple	25

Mid-morning snack

1 rice-cake	28
1 teaspoon low-calorie jam	10

Lunch

Hard-boiled egg and cress sandwich with wholemeal bread	245

Mid-afternoon snack

2oz (55g) raw carrot	13

Dinner

*Curried beef pancakes (wholemeal)	385
*Bean and sweetcorn salad	25

Dessert

*Bran and sultana bread	160

TOTAL CALORIES	1,014

FACTS

● Some foods rich in fibre contain phytic acid. This substance blocks the absorption of zinc, calcium, copper, and vitamin B_6 from other foods in the diet. This is a distinct disadvantage of some fibre-rich diets.

● The highest sources of phytic acid are, in descending order, wheat, bran, wheat germ, brown rice, corn bran, oats, beans and peas. The amount in carrots and other vegetables is very small.

Daily chart

Today's weight _____

Symptoms _____

_____

_____

_____

_____

_____

REVIEW YOUR PROGRESS

If you have experienced adverse symptoms this week, you may not be feeling as well as you did at the end of last week. You may find that your weight has fluctuated or even gone up. *Do not be discouraged* if this has occurred. Simply record the suspect foods, discard them from your diet, and continue without them.

If you are not feeling as well as you did at the beginning of the week, go back to the Stage I diet for two or three days; your weight should fall again if it rose during this week.

Don't forget to record positive foods

As well as making a note of any foods that have caused reactions, keep a note of all the foods that you feel happy about eating, i.e. those that have not caused you any problems or any weight gain.

If you were able to eat wheat or any of the other grains this week without any ill-effects, you will be able to include this food in your diet in Stage III. That is why it is vital that you keep accurate records. *You will not be eating even positive foods from the 'wheat' week again at any time in Stage II. It is essential to remember this.*

WEEK-ENDING CHART Stage II				
Date				
Total weight loss this week	Suspect foods discovered	Safe foods discovered	General degree of well-being*	Any other comments or observations
Weight at beginning of week				
Weight at end of week				
Change in weight				

*Score degree of well-being
Very well 3   Well 2   Fair 1   Unwell 0

RECIPES

Fish crumble

Serves 2   Calories per serving 385

7oz (200g) cod fillet
1 carrot, sliced
3oz (85g) green beans, sliced
3 fresh tomatoes, peeled and sliced
1 small onion, thinly sliced
1 clove garlic, finely chopped
½ teaspoon basil
1 teaspoon parsley
Fresh black pepper
1 tablespoon cornflour
1 tablespoon water

For the crumble:
1oz (30g) wholemeal flour
1oz (30g) plain flour
4 teaspoons margarine

1. Place the garlic, onion, carrot, beans, basil, parsley and tomatoes in a saucepan.
2. Remove the skin from the fish, and cut the fish into strips, about 1½ inches (3.5cm) across. Add to the saucepan, season with pepper.
3. Bring this mixture to boil, cover, and reduce the heat. Simmer for 12–15 minutes.
4. Blend the cornflour to a paste with water, stir into the fish mixture, and bring to the boil. Transfer the mixture to a deep, oven-proof dish.
5. Make the crumble topping, rubbing the two flours and margarine together until the mixture resembles breadcrumbs.
6. Sprinkle the crumble over the fish and bake for 20–25 minutes at 180°C/350°F/Gas Mark 4.

Chicken and sweetcorn lasagne

Serves 5   Calories per serving 350

2 × 7oz (200g) chicken breasts
  chopped into 1-inch (2.5cm)
  pieces
1 small onion, sliced
1 small carrot, sliced
1 bay leaf
1 teaspoon mixed herbs
2 tablespoons sweetcorn
4oz (115g) wholewheat lasagne
1¼oz (40g) skimmed milk powder
2oz (55g) low-fat spread
2oz (55g) flour
Freshly ground black pepper to taste
3 tablespoons wholewheat
  breadcrumbs

1. Place the chicken breast pieces
   without skin in a saucepan with
   the carrot and onion. Add the bay
   leaf and mixed herbs. Add
   enough water to just cover the
   chicken and bring to the boil.
   Cover the pan and simmer gently
   for 25 minutes.
2. Place the wholewheat lasagne in
   plenty of water and cook for 5
   minutes less than the
   recommended time. Rinse under
   the cold water tap.
3. Remove the chicken from the
   saucepan and drain off the juice.
   Discard carrot and onion. Make
   the liquid up to 1 pint (570ml) by
   adding either vegetable juice or
   water. Place in a saucepan with
   the skimmed milk powder, low-
   fat spread and flour. Bring to the
   boil, whisking all the time, and
   then simmer for 2 minutes. Add
   freshly ground pepper.
4. Stir the chicken and sweetcorn
   into the sauce. Spread one-third
   of the sauce over the base and
   add one layer of half the lasagne.
   Spread half of the remaining
   sauce over the lasagne. Add the
   other half of lasagne and again
   another layer of sauce. Sprinkle
   the breadcrumbs over the top and
   bake for 30 minutes at 190°C/
   375°F/Gas Mark 5.

Lentil rissoles

Serves 2   Calories per serving 290

4oz (115g) split red lentils
½ teaspoon (2.5ml) ground cumin
½ teaspoon (2.5ml) ground
coriander
¼ teaspoon (1.25ml) chilli powder
Freshly ground black pepper
1 egg, size 3
8floz (225ml) water
2 level teaspoons butter
Wholemeal breadcrumbs

1. Wash the lentils under cold running water. Drain and place in a saucepan with water. Cover and bring to the boil. Simmer gently for 30 minutes until water has been absorbed. Check frequently, and add extra water if the water is absorbed too quickly, so the lentils do not burn.
2. Melt the butter in the saucepan over a low heat. Stir in the cumin, coriander and chilli powder for 1–2 minutes, stirring constantly. Then add the lentils and season with freshly ground black pepper.
3. Separate the egg, and add the yolk to the lentils. Mix well, then leave to cool.
4. Divide into 4, and shape into 4 cakes.
5. Brush the cakes with the egg white and then press on the wholemeal breadcrumbs.
6. Place on a baking sheet and bake for 15 minutes at 200°C/400°F/ Gas Mark 6.

Pizza toast

Serves 1   Calories 280

2 slices of wholemeal toast

For the topping:
1 teaspoon oil
½ onion, chopped
1 tablespoon tomato purée
1 small garlic clove, crushed
2 large tomatoes, skinned and
  chopped
¼ small green pepper, chopped
2 sardines, canned in tomato sauce,
  drained
½ teaspoon mixed herbs

1. Heat the oil and fry the onions and garlic for 2–3 minutes.
2. Add the tomatoes, mixed herbs, tomato purée and peppers.
3. Simmer for a further 2–3 minutes.
4. Chop the sardines and add to sauce gently. Stir until the sardines are heated through.
5. Cover each piece of toast with sauce. Grill gently for 1 minute.

Wholewheat spaghetti with ham and spinach sauce

Serves 4   Calories per serving 275

6oz (170g) cooked, lean ham,
  chopped into small pieces
1 medium onion, chopped
8oz (225g) frozen chopped spinach
½ pint (285ml) boiling water
½ level teaspoon mixed dried herbs
3floz (85ml) cold water
1 level tablespoon cornflour
2oz (55g) skimmed milk powder
4oz (115g) wholewheat spaghetti

1. Place the onions in a saucepan with the spinach, boiling water and mixed herbs.
2. Cover the pan and simmer gently for 5 minutes.
3. Purée the onions and spinach in a liquidizer or food processor.
4. Blend the skimmed milk powder and cornflour with cold water. Place in a saucepan with the spinach purée and bring to the boil, stirring constantly. Simmer for 1–2 minutes.
5. Meanwhile boil the spaghetti until just tender, 12–15 minutes.
6. Add the ham to the sauce with freshly ground black pepper, and heat for 1–2 minutes.
7. Drain the spaghetti and divide between four plates and top with sauce.

Curried beef pancakes

Serves 4   Calories per serving 385

4oz (115g) plain flour
1 egg, size 3
½ pint (285ml) skimmed milk
1 teaspoon sunflower oil

For the filling:
12oz (340g) minced beef
1 medium onion
2 level tablespoons (30ml) cornflour
2 level teaspoons (10ml) curry
  powder
4 level tablespoons (60ml) skimmed
  milk powder
2 tablespoons (30ml) tomato purée
1 pint (570ml) water
4 level tablespoons (60ml) mango
  chutney
2 level tablespoons (30ml) apricot
  jam
2 tablespoons (30ml) Weight
  Watchers beef soup
Pepper to taste

1. Make a batter with the flour, egg and milk. Use a small greased frying pan and make the pancakes. The mixture will make approximately 8 thin pancakes.
2. Mix the milk powder, half the curry powder and cornflour with enough water to make a smooth paste. Mix with the remaining water and pour into a saucepan. Add to this the apricot jam, the mango chutney and the Weight Watchers beef soup. Bring gently to the boil and then simmer gently for 2 minutes. Now put this to one side.
3. Chop the onion finely. Brown the mince in a frying pan, strain off the excess fat and add the chopped onions, the remaining curry powder, the tomato purée, and about one-third of the curry sauce. Stir well. Simmer in a covered pan for 15 minutes, stirring occasionally. Add a little water if necessary to prevent the mixture drying.
4. Fill each of the pancakes with curry mixture and roll them up. Place them in a covered oven-proof dish, and then into the oven for 12 minutes at 190°C/375°F/Gas Mark 5.
5. Heat the remaining curry sauce and pour a little over each pancake as they are served.

Beef and spinach pasta

Serves 4　　Calories per serving 310

12oz (340g) frozen chopped spinach
12oz (340g) very lean minced beef
5 medium tomatoes, skinned and
　chopped
1 tablespoon flour
1 green pepper, chopped
4oz (115g) sweetcorn
6oz (170g) wholewheat pasta shells
1 teaspoon mixed dried herbs
1 tablespoon tomato purée
Freshly ground black pepper

1. Cook the spinach as directed on
   the packet. Place in a sieve and
   press lightly with the back of a
   spoon to remove excess water.
2. Brown the mince in a frying pan.
   Drain off and discard fat. Stir the
   flour into the mince.
3. Add the tomato purée, green
   pepper, tomatoes, herbs and
   sweetcorn. Season with black
   pepper.
4. Cover and simmer for 15–20
   minutes.
5. Boil the wholewheat pasta shells
   as directed on the packet.
6. Add the spinach to the sauce and
   heat through for 1–2 minutes
   before serving.

Turkey in wholemeal breadcrumbs

Serves 1　　Calories 254

4oz (115g) turkey breast
1 egg
1 tablespoon wholemeal
　breadcrumbs

1. Whisk the egg and brush over the
   turkey breast.
2. Place wholemeal breadcrumbs in
   shallow bowl and dip the turkey
   breast both sides until coated.
3. Place on aluminium foil and grill
   for 15–20 minutes, turning
   occasionally until cooked.

NB: Salad recipes appear in Stage I, pages 142–5

Lemon fruit roll

Approximately 10 slices   Calories per serving 96

3 eggs
1 level tablespoon (15ml)
  concentrated apple juice
½ teaspoon (2.5ml) sunflower oil
2oz (55g) white self-raising flour
2 tablespoons (30ml) hot water
4 tablespoons (60ml) lemon curd
4 rings of canned pineapple in
  natural juice
Rind of 1 lemon, grated

1. Line a swiss roll tin (8×11 inches/20×28cm) with greaseproof paper and brush lightly with the oil.
2. Separate the eggs and whisk the yolks with grated lemon rind and the concentrated apple juice until light and creamy.
3. Sieve the flour and fold into the egg mixture with the water.
4. Whisk the egg white until stiff and then fold gently into the mixture.
5. Gently place the mixture in the prepared swiss roll tin and bake for 12–15 minutes at 200°C/400°F/Gas Mark 6.
6. Turn out onto a sheet of greaseproof paper and trim the edges.
7. Roll up with the paper inside and leave to cool.
8. Unroll the swiss roll gently and spread with the lemon curd and chopped pineapple pieces.
9. Roll up again and place on a serving dish.

Pancakes with lemon and sugar

Serves 4   Calories per serving 150

Make 8 wholemeal pancakes as in the recipe on page 169, then add lemon and sugar to taste.

Alternative fillings

Put one teaspoon (5ml) of low-calorie jam in the centre of each pancake and roll up *or*
Add one tablespoon (15ml) of stewed fruit and roll up.

Apple Charlotte

Serves 4   Calories per serving 155

1 level teaspoon (5ml) low-fat spread
1lb (455g) cooking apples
4 tablespoons (60ml) honey
3oz (85g) wholemeal breadcrumbs
4 tablespoons (60ml) already diluted
  apple juice
¼ level teaspoon (1.25ml) ground
  ginger

1. Lightly grease 4 individual oven-proof dishes with low-fat spread.
2. Slice the apples and arrange half equally between the dishes.
3. Top with half the honey and sprinkle on half the breadcrumbs.
4. Repeat the layers until they have used up the ingredients.
5. Add on the apple juice and sprinkle on the ginger. Place in oven at 180°C/ 350°F/Gas Mark 4 for about 1 hour until the apples are tender and topping is crisp.

Sponge cake

Makes 8 slices   Calories per slice 140

3oz (85g) wholemeal flour
3 eggs, size 3
4oz (115g) caster sugar
3 level tablespoons (45ml) low-calorie jam

1. Line the base of 2×7-inch (17.5cm) sandwich tins with greaseproof paper, brush the insides with oil, and dust with a teaspoon of the flour.
2. Place the eggs and sugar in a large basin and stand over a saucepan of simmering water.
3. Whisk until light and fluffy and then remove the basin from the pan.
4. Sift the flour over the surface of the mixture and fold in gently.
5. Spread the mixture evenly between the two tins and bake in the oven at 190°C/375°F/Gas Mark 5 for 25 minutes or until well risen.
6. Cool on a wire rack.
7. Sandwich together with the jam.

Carrot and date cake

Makes approximately 16 slices   Calories per slice 115

2oz (55g) low-calorie margarine
6 tablespoons (90ml) honey
¼ teaspoon (1.25ml) sunflower oil
4oz (115g) carrots, peeled
4oz (115g) dates, stoned
6oz (170g) plain granary flour
1 level teaspoon (5ml) bicarbonate of soda
½ level teaspoon (2.5ml) baking powder
½ level teaspoon (2.5ml) cinnamon
1 egg, size 3
4floz (115ml) skimmed milk
3 tablespoons (45ml) unsweetened orange juice

1. Line a 6-inch (15cm) square tin with greaseproof paper and brush with a little oil.
2. Place the margarine and honey in a small pan and warm until it has melted.
3. Finely grate the carrots and chop the dates.
4. Mix together the flour, bicarbonate of soda, baking powder and cinnamon.
5. Beat the egg with the milk and orange juice until blended.
6. Add the egg mixture to the honey and margarine mixture.
7. Stir all the ingredients together gently until thoroughly mixed.
8. Pour the mixture into the tins and bake for 1 hour.
9. Cool on a wire rack.

Bran and sultana bread

Makes 12 slices   Calories per serving 160

3oz (85g) of All-Bran
4oz (115g) caster sugar
½ pint (285ml) skimmed milk
6oz (170g) wholemeal self-raising flour
8oz (225g) sultanas
1 level teaspoon (5ml) baking powder
¼ teaspoon (1.25ml) of oil

1. Place the All-Bran, sultanas, caster sugar and milk in a bowl.
2. Stir the mixture, cover and refrigerate for several hours.
3. Sieve flour and baking powder and stir into the soaked mixture.
4. Line a 2lb (1kg) loaf tin and brush with the oil.
5. Turn the loaf mixture into the tin and level the top.
6. Bake at 190°C/375°F/Gas Mark 5 for about 1¼ hours (until an inserted skewer comes out clean).
7. Cool on a wire rack.

Apple scones

Makes 8 scones   Calories per scone 170

5oz (140g) plain white flour
4oz (115g) plain wholemeal flour
2oz (55g) caster sugar
1oz (30g) butter
8oz (225g) cooking apples
4floz (115ml) skimmed milk
4 level teaspoons (20ml) baking powder
¼ teaspoon (1.25ml) sunflower oil
¼ level teaspoon (1.25ml) ground cinnamon
¼ level teaspoon (1.25ml) ground mixed spice

1. Sieve 4oz (115g) of the white flour with the baking powder, cinnamon and mixed spice.
2. Add the wholemeal flour and sugar.
3. Rub in the butter.
4. Wash, peel, core and then grate the apples and stir into the flour mixture together with the milk to make a soft droppy dough.
5. Roll out into a circle ½-inch (1cm) thick and then cut into 8 scones.
6. Brush a baking sheet with the oil and arrange the scones on it.
7. Bake at 220°C/425°F/Gas Mark 7 for 10–15 minutes until golden brown.
8. Cool on a wire rack.

PACKED LUNCHES

	Calories		Calories
Wholemeal pitta bread, filled with 2oz (55g) shredded lettuce, 1 sliced tomato, 1 slice of onion, 4 slices of cucumber	184	Sardines (in tomato sauce) 3oz (85g)	150
		Chicken breast (no skin) 3oz (85g)	120

You can add to this:

You can use any lean meat.

Tuna (canned in brine) 3oz (85g)	90
Salmon (canned) 3oz (85g)	131
Pilchards (canned in tomato sauce)	106

Sandwich — again you can use any of the above fillings: two slices of wholemeal bread spread with two teaspoons of low-fat spread   190

SNACKS

As Stage I (page 100), or:

1 slice wholemeal toast   70

ELIZABETH MARSHALL

Elizabeth is a 27-year-old midwife who considers she has been at least a stone (14lb/6.5kg) overweight since she was aged 16. She also suffered with abdominal bloating, headaches, irritability, depression and severe cravings for sweet foods.

'I used to get desperate for chocolate. On my worst days I would eat five or six bars of chocolate. I tried calorie counting and also the Cambridge Diet. I could not stick to any diet for very long because of the chocolate cravings.

'I lost 1½ stones on the WNAS programme. I had to cut down on dairy products and grains. It took me three months to lose the weight, but I felt so well on the programme and was never hungry. I found I could eat as much of the unrestricted foods as I wanted and I still steadily lost weight.

'I have experienced long-term changes as a result of the WNAS programme. I had been struggling with my marriage for years largely because of my mood swings. As I feel so well now I have been able to sort out the problems with my husband and we now feel that we have got back the relationship we got married to share.

'I am generally more positive and interested in life. I now have a regular exercise programme which I enjoy and I am a trim 1½ stones lighter which makes all the difference to how I feel about myself.'

22
Week 2 —
dairy produce

During this second week of Stage II you will be putting dairy produce back into your diet: extra cow's milk, yogurt, cheese, butter, and cream. You should not be eating any of the grain products from last week, whether they suited you or not.

Use the suggested menus as a guide. You can vary the menu according to your taste within the restrictions mentioned, but make sure you do not exceed your daily calorie allowance.

Again, you must complete the chart daily. If you experience reactions to any dairy produce then you must record these and exclude the food again from your diet.

Remember, if you get a mild reaction, you will need to proceed with caution until you can tell whether that food or food group is causing you to feel less well or less able to lose weight than you were at the end of Stage I.

WEEK 2 — DAY 1

Breakfast	Calories
1oz (30g) Rice Krispies	105
3floz (95ml) skimmed milk	28

Mid-morning snack

3½oz (100g) Shape yogurt	40

Lunch

2oz (55g) cheese on toast (slimmer's bread)	276
½ tomato sliced on top	4

Mid-afternoon snack

1oz (30g) Shape low-fat Cheddar cheese	73

Dinner

*Poached halibut in parsley sauce	250
4oz (115g) potatoes	90
4oz (115g) carrots	21
4oz (115g) spring greens	11

Dessert

*Gooseberry mousse	100
TOTAL CALORIES	**998**

FACTS

● On average, some 10 per cent of daily calorie intake comes from milk, a further 4 per cent from cream and cheese, 7 per cent from butter.

● Dairy products make up over 20 per cent of our calories and they also provide over 20 per cent of our protein intake and much of our calcium.

Daily chart

Today's weight _____

Symptoms _____

_____

_____

_____

_____

_____

WEEK 2 — DAY 2

Breakfast	Calories
1 egg and cheese (½oz/15g) omelette	137
1 slice of slimmer's toast or 2 rice-cakes	56
1 teaspoon low-calorie spread	25
1 teaspoon low-calorie jam	10

Mid-morning snack

3oz (85g) stick celery	6

Lunch

4oz (115g) tuna in brine (drained)	150
Jacket potato with 1oz (30g) sour cream	145

Mid-afternoon snack

2oz (55g) raw carrot	13

Dinner

*Spinach and egg bake	240
*Cauliflower and carrot salad	30
2oz (55g) brown rice	66

Dessert

*Passion fruit fool	135

TOTAL CALORIES	1,013

FACTS

● Butter provides 200 calories per ounce; half a pound of butter is almost a day's calorie intake for an adult female! It contains good amounts of vitamins A and D, but no minerals and no protein and is almost 100 per cent fat.

● There are different types of fats: saturated fats, which are found mainly in animal produce, and unsaturated fats, which are found mainly in vegetable produce. Both are important and concentrated sources of energy but some unsaturated fats are needed for good health.

Daily chart

Today's weight _____

Symptoms _____

_____

_____

_____

_____

_____

WEEK 2 — DAY 3

Breakfast	**Calories**
1oz (30g) cornflakes	104
3floz (85ml) skimmed milk	28

Mid-morning snack

3½oz (100g) Shape yogurt	40
1 apple, grated	50

Lunch

*Steamed whiting in cheese sauce	287
*Green salad	32

Mid-afternoon snack

1oz (30g) Shape low-fat cheese	73

Dinner

4oz (115g) grilled lamb chop	222
4oz (115g) cauliflower	10
4oz (115g) carrots	21
4oz (115g) boiled potatoes	90

Dessert

Yogurt ice-cream	50

TOTAL CALORIES	1,007

FACTS

● A diet high in saturated (animal) fats and low in poly-unsaturates increases the risk of heart disease. Mediterranean countries, where there is a lower intake of saturated fat and a more balanced intake of unsaturated fat, have a lower heart disease risk.

● A diet low in saturated fats and with a higher percentage of polyunsaturates (just like the diet you were on) has been shown to help premenstrual breast tenderness. It may also help reduce the risk of breast cancer in the future.

Daily chart

Today's weight _____

Symptoms _____

_____

_____

_____

_____

_____

WEEK 2 — DAY 4

Breakfast	Calories
1oz (30g) Rice Krispies	105
3floz (85ml) skimmed milk	28
1 orange, chopped	50

Mid-morning snack	
4oz (115g) raw carrots	26

Lunch	
*Haddock kedgeree (unsmoked)	290
*Green salad	32

Mid-afternoon snack	
1 apple	50

Dinner	
*Beef Stroganoff	275
2oz (55g) brown rice	66
4oz (55g) broccoli	20
4oz (115g) French beans	8

Dessert	
*Iced stuffed apples	60

| TOTAL CALORIES | 1,010 |

FACTS

● Some unsaturated fats are chemically altered in the process of being made into margarine. This process, called hydrogenation, makes the fat more solid, giving us hard rather than soft margarine. The hard, hydrogenated margarines do not carry the health benefits of polyunsaturated margarines, and are best avoided on this diet programme.

● Fish and chips, and other fast foods, are usually cooked in palm oil or palm oil blends. They are too low in polyunsaturates.

Daily chart

Today's weight _____

Symptoms _____

_____

_____

_____

_____

WEEK 2 — DAY 5

Breakfast	Calories
1oz (30g) Rice Krispies	105
3floz (85ml) skimmed milk	28
½ apple, grated	25

Mid-morning snack

1oz (30g) Shape low-fat cheese	73
3oz (85g) stick of celery	6

Lunch

Jacket potato	96
4oz (115g) cottage cheese and 1 orange mixed together	158

Mid-afternoon snack

1 rice-cake with 1 teaspoon low-calorie jam	38

Dinner

4oz (115g) roast turkey breast	148
4oz (115g) cauliflower in *Cheese sauce	205
4oz (115g) spinach	34
4oz (115g) carrots	21

Dessert

*Melon ice-cream	65
TOTAL CALORIES	**1,002**

FACTS

● Diets high in saturated fats are often, but not necessarily, high in cholesterol. The saturated fat in a diet, more importantly, stimulates the liver to produce more cholesterol in a form that is easily deposited onto the linings of the arteries.

● On average some 40 per cent of our daily calories are derived from dietary fats. Several expert committees now recommend that this is reduced to 30–35 per cent of calorie intake. This means reducing your fat intake to three-quarters of its current level.

Daily chart

Today's weight _____

Symptoms _____

_____

_____

_____

_____

_____

WEEK 2 — DAY 6

Breakfast	Calories
2 scrambled eggs	160
2 grilled tomatoes	16
1 slice of slimmer's bread	40

Mid-morning snack

2oz (55g) raw carrot	13

Lunch

3oz (85g) Edam cheese	228
*Ginger and carrot salad	36
1 tablespoon (15ml) low- calorie dressing	25

Mid-afternoon snack

3½oz (100g) Shape yogurt	40

Dinner

*Salmon and cheese roll	195
4oz (115g) boiled potatoes	90
4oz (115g) spring greens	11
4oz (115g) runner beans	21

Dessert

*Blackberries with hazelnut cheese	140
TOTAL CALORIES	**1,015**

FACTS

● Fat delays the emptying of the stomach, thus producing a feeling of satisfaction after a meal. However, because fatty foods contain lots of calories in a small space, it is easy to eat such foods quickly, and potentially to put on weight.

● Fish oils contain a special type of polyunsaturated oils and good sources of these are mackerel, herring, salmon, sardines and tuna. Such oils may help to lower the risks of heart disease by reducing the stickiness of blood that can lead to a heart attack.

Daily chart

Today's weight _____

Symptoms _____

_____

_____

_____

_____

_____

WEEK 2 — DAY 7

Breakfast	Calories
1¼oz (35g) rasher of lean bacon (grilled)	80
1 poached egg (size 3)	80
1 piece of slimmer's bread	40

Mid-morning snack

3½oz (100g) Shape yogurt	40
½ apple, grated	25

Lunch

Steamed vegetables with *Chive and cheese sauce	195
Jacket potato	96

Mid-afternoon snack

1 piece of fruit	50

Dinner

4oz (115g) roast beef (lean)	192
4oz (115g) marrow	8
4oz (115g) spinach	34
4oz (115g) boiled potatoes	90

Dessert

*Grapefruit sorbet	85
TOTAL CALORIES	1,015

FACTS

● Allergies to cow's milk protein are quite common in childhood and present a number of problems, including eczema, asthma or wheezing, infantile colic, hyperactive behaviour, nettle-rash (urticaria), constipation, diarrhoea, and even bleeding from the bowel, catarrh, and recurrent ear infection or 'glue ears'.

● In adults, milk can cause asthma, rhinitis (a stuffy or runny nose), urticaria, diarrhoea, and other bowel problems.

Daily chart

Today's weight _____

Symptoms _____

_____

_____

_____

_____

WEEK-ENDING CHART
Stage II

Date

Total weight loss this week	Suspect foods discovered	Safe foods discovered	General degree of well-being*	Any other comments or observations
Weight at beginning of week				
Weight at end of week				
Change in weight				

*Score degree of well-being
Very well 3   Well 2   Fair 1   Unwell 0

REVIEW YOUR PROGRESS

After eating dairy produce for a week, you should have a pretty good idea about whether it suited you or not. If you sailed through this week without any problems, then all you need do is mark on your end of week chart 'no symptoms'.

If you have experienced an adverse reaction this week, then you will have to discard some of the dairy products from your diet. Make sure your records reflect this before you move on to Week 3 of Stage II.

Don't forget to record your weight loss for the week, and to make a note of the foods you discovered you felt well on. Also remember that you will not be using dairy products next week, but you will be introducing foods that contain yeast and alcohol.

RECIPES

Spinach and egg bake

Serves 2   Calories per serving 240

1oz (30g) low-fat cheese, grated
12oz (340g) frozen chopped spinach
2 eggs
8 teaspoons (40ml) single cream
Freshly ground black pepper to taste

1. Grease two 4-inch oven-proof dishes.
2. Boil spinach, following instructions on packet. Press in a sieve to drain excess water.
3. Divide the spinach between the two dishes and make a deep well in the centre. Break an egg into each well.
4. Spoon 4 teaspoons of cream over each egg and season well with pepper.
5. Bake at 180°C/350°F/Gas Mark 4 for 20 minutes.
6. Remove from oven, sprinkle with cheese and grill for 1–2 minutes. Serve immediately.

Steamed whiting in cheese sauce

Serves 2   Calories per serving 287

2×5oz (140g) whiting fillets
Cheese sauce (see recipe page 187)
1oz (30g) Shape low-fat cheese, grated
1 tomato, sliced
Freshly ground black pepper

1. Stream the whiting fillets over a pan of boiling water in a metal colander for about 10–15 minutes, until the fish flakes easily.
2. Place into a heat-proof serving dish and cover with cheese sauce.
3. Place tomato slices over each fillet, sprinkle with low-fat cheese and grill for 1–2 minutes.

Cheese sauce

Serves 4   Calories per serving 100

½ pint (285ml) skimmed milk
4oz (115g) low-fat cheese
1oz (30g) plain flour
½oz (15g) margarine

1. Melt the fat in a saucepan, add the flour and cook for a few minutes stirring constantly.
2. Slowly add the milk, again stirring, and cook over a low heat until the sauce thickens.
3. Take off the heat and add the cheese, stirring until the mixture is smooth.

Variations
Chive and cheese sauce: add finely chopped or snipped chives just before serving.

Haddock kedgeree

Serves 2   Calories per serving 290

6oz (170g) unsmoked haddock, filleted and skinned
3oz (85g) brown rice
1 hard-boiled egg, chopped
½ green pepper, chopped
1 small onion, finely chopped
2 tablespoons low-fat natural yogurt
Freshly ground black pepper to taste
2 slices of lemon
1 sprig parsley

1. Cover the fish with water in a shallow pan. Heat gently and poach for about 8–10 minutes.
2. Remove the fish and flake.
3. Boil the rice in the poaching water left in the pan for about 10 minutes. See cooking instructions on the rice packet. You may need to add extra water.
4. Drain rice, stir in the fish, egg, onion, pepper, parsley and yogurt and mix well. Heat gently, stirring all the time.
5. Season with pepper and serve garnished with lemon.

Beef Stroganoff

Serves 4   Calories per serving 275

1lb (455g) fillet of beef
1 medium onion, finely sliced
4oz (115g) red pepper, chopped
2 teaspoons of oil
1oz (30g) butter
½ beef stock cube
¼ pint (140ml) boiling water
1 level teaspoon tomato purée
6 level tablespoons (90ml) soured
  cream
Freshly ground black pepper to taste

1. Heat half the oil and half the butter in a non-stick frying pan. Add the onion, and cook over a low heat, stirring frequently, until soft.
2. Stir in the peppers.
3. Dissolve the stock cube in the water, stir in the tomato purée, then add to the pan. Boil rapidly until the liquid is reduced to about 2floz (60ml/4 tablespoons). Tip the reduced liquid into a bowl and set aside.
4. Heat the remaining oil and butter in the pan and add the meat, which should all fit in the pan easily in a single layer. If necessary, cook it in two batches. Cook over a fairly high heat until the outsides are browned — about 3 minutes each side. Shake and toss the pan frequently as the meat cooks. Add the vegetable mixture and heat through. Add the soured cream and season. Heat through but do not allow to boil.
5. Serve immediately.

Poached halibut with parsley sauce

Serves 6   Calories per serving 250

6×6oz (170g) halibut steaks
2 tablespoons freshly chopped
  parsley
1 small leek, chopped
1 carrot, peeled and chopped
3 tablespoons (45ml) lemon juice
5floz (140ml) water

1. Place the chopped vegetables and 1 tablespoon of parsley over the bottom of a large pan. Add the steaks on top with the lemon juice and water.
2. Bring to the boil, cover and simmer for about 10 minutes.
3. Transfer the halibut to a dish and keep warm.
4. Bring the liquid and vegetables back to the boil and simmer for a further 5 minutes.
5. Blend the vegetables to a purée and return to saucepan.
6. Add the remaining tablespoon of parsley and reduce liquid until it has thickened.
7. Pour liquid over halibut steaks and serve.

Salmon and cheese roll

Serves 2   Calories per serving 195

4×1oz (30g) slices smoked salmon
3oz (85g) cottage cheese
3oz (85g) curd cheese
½ apple, shredded
1 teaspoon lemon juice
Black pepper to taste
2oz (55g) lettuce, chopped
2 lemon slices

1. Mix the cottage and curd cheese with lemon juice and shredded apple. Season with black pepper.
2. Lay each smoked salmon slice on a flat surface and spread with the cheese mixture. Roll up (like a swiss roll).
3. Garnish with lemon slice and serve on a bed of lettuce.

NB: Salad recipes appear in Stage I.

Gooseberry mousse

Serves 4   Calories per serving 100

1lb (455g) gooseberries
1 tablespoon lime juice
½ pint (285ml) unsweetened apple
   purée
3 tablespoons (45ml) natural yogurt
1 tablespoon (15ml) clear honey
Concentrated apple juice
3 teaspoons (15ml) powdered
   gelatine
2 tablespoons (30ml) water
1 egg white

1. Prepare the gooseberries and stew
   lightly. Add concentrated apple
   juice to taste.
2. Blend the gooseberries and lime
   juice in the liquidizer and make
   the mixture up to ½ pint by
   adding water.
3. Mix the gooseberries and the
   apple purée together, and add the
   honey and yogurt.
4. Put the gelatine and water into a
   small bowl. Stand the bowl over a
   pan or in hot water and stir until
   the gelatine has dissolved.
5. Stir the gelatine mixture into the
   fruit purée.
6. Whisk the egg white until stiff
   and fold lightly into the
   gooseberry and apple mixture.
7. Spoon into 4 dessert glasses and
   chill for at least 2–3 hours before
   serving.

Passion fruit fool

Serves 4   Calories per serving 135

6 ripe passion fruit (or a substitute fruit)
¼ pint (5floz/140ml) skimmed milk
¼ pint (5floz/140ml) natural yogurt
2 teaspoons cornflour
2 tablespoons (30ml) water
1 tablespoon (15ml) clear honey

1. Halve the passion fruit and scoop the fruit pulp into a bowl.
2. Gently heat the skimmed milk.
3. Blend the cornflour and water into a smooth paste and then stir into the hot milk. Stir over the heat until the sauce has thickened, and remove to cool slightly.
4. Stir the yogurt and honey into the sauce and leave until cool.
5. Combine the sauce and the passion fruit pulp and then spoon the mixture into serving dishes.
6. Chill for 3–4 hours and serve from the refrigerator.

Yogurt ice-cream

Serves 4   Calories per serving 50

8oz (225g) raspberries, plums, peaches or other soft fruit
10oz (285g) natural yogurt
1 teaspoon (5ml) concentrated apple juice to sweeten
Mint sprig to decorate

1. Wash and prepare the fruit as necessary, and purée it in the liquidizer with all the remaining ingredients.
2. Spoon the mixture into a freezer container with a lid and place in the freezer for 2–3 hours until semi-frozen.
3. Remove the mixture from the freezer, add the yogurt and whisk well, then freeze until firm.
4. Place the yogurt ice-cream in the refrigerator 30 minutes before serving to allow it to soften.
5. Scoop the ice-cream into chilled dessert dishes and decorate with fruit or mint.

Iced stuffed apples

Serves 4   Calories per serving 60

2 medium cooking apples
4 dessert apples
2 egg yolks
1 egg white
3 tablespoons (45ml) natural yogurt
2 tablespoons sultanas
4 tablespoons (60ml) lemon juice

1. Stew the cooking apples with half the lemon juice in a covered saucepan.
2. Beat the egg yolks, add to the fruit and allow to cool.
3. Mix the yogurt with the cooled purée and then pour into a shallow dish and freeze until firm at the edges.
4. Cut a thin slice from each dessert apple (about ½-inch/1cm) to be used as lids.
5. Hollow out the centre of each apple carefully, removing the flesh and the core but leaving a shell about ¼-inch (5mm) thick.
6. Brush the inside of the apples with the remaining lemon juice.
7. Spoon the semi-frozen apple mixture into a bowl and beat until smooth.
8. Whisk the egg white until stiff and fold lightly into the apple mixture, adding the sultanas.
9. Spoon the apple mixture into the hollow apples and replace the lids. Place in the freezer until firm.
10. Allow a few minutes for the apples to stand outside the freezer so that the centres have a chance to soften slightly before you serve them.

Blackberries with hazelnut cheese

Serves 6   Calories per serving 140

1½lb (680g) blackberries (fresh or frozen)
1 tablespoon soft dark brown sugar
2oz (55g) hazelnuts
1 teaspoon caster sugar
6 petit suisse cheeses
½ tablespoon (7.5ml) tropical fruit juice

1. Clean and prepare the blackberries. Mix with the brown sugar and tropical fruit juice.
2. Toast the hazelnuts in a frying pan and add the caster sugar when the nuts are brown. Shake the pan continuously to coat the nuts in the melting sugar and set aside on a plate to cool.
3. Grind the caramel-coated nuts and spread them out on a large sheet of greaseproof paper.
4. Roll each petit suisse in the crushed nuts, gently pressing the nuts onto the surface of the cheese.
5. Place the individual cheeses on a plate and then into the refrigerator to set.
6. When you are about to serve, place the individual cheese balls in dessert glasses and surround each one with the berries.

Grapefruit sorbet

Serves 4   Calories per serving 85

2 grapefruits
¾ pint (425ml) water
Concentrated apple juice
3 tablespoons (45ml) natural yogurt
2 egg whites
Peeled grapefruit segments for
    decoration

1. Thinly pare the rind from the grapefruit and place the grapefruit rind and water into a pan. Simmer gently for 8 minutes and strain into a bowl.
2. Cut the fruit in half and squeeze out the juice.
3. Add the grapefruit juice to the liquid from the grapefruit rind into a bowl and add apple juice to taste.
4. Pour the grapefruit liquid into a shallow freezer container and freeze until semi-frozen.
5. Turn the semi-frozen grapefruit mixture into a bowl and beat to break up the ice crystals.
6. Mix in the yogurt.
7. Whisk the egg white until stiff and fold into the grapefruit and yogurt mixture gently.
8. Return to the freezer until firm.
9. Scoop the sorbet into dessert glasses and decorate with peeled grapefruit segments.

Melon ice-cream

Serves 4   Calories per serving 65

1 medium melon (ogen or similar if
   you can get it)
½ pint (285ml) plain yogurt
Concentrated apple juice to sweeten
   if necessary
Melon balls to decorate

1. Half the melon, scoop out the
   seeds and then scoop out the
   melon flesh and place in the
   liquidizer.
2. Liquidize the melon flesh and
   mix with the yogurt and
   concentrated apple juice as
   needed.
3. Place the melon and yogurt
   mixture in a shallow dish and
   freeze until firm.
4. Scoop the melon ice-cream into
   dessert glasses and decorate with
   melon balls.

PACKED LUNCHES

Use any of the salads from the salad
recipes, adding:
Cheddar cheese
        2oz (55g)=Calories 229
Lancashire cheese
        2oz (55g)=Calories 202
Edam cheese
        2oz (55g)=Calories 180
Cottage cheese
        4oz (115g)=Calories 108

You can add yogurt as a salad dressing,
or have it after your salad. Most low-
fat yogurts are about 40 calories per
3½oz (100g) — less for natural.

Rice-cakes with cheese and tomato
topping — 1oz (30g) cheese sliced on
top of each rice-cake, 1 slice of tomato
or onion on top: Calories per rice-cake
145.

SNACKS

As Stage I (page 100), or:

3½oz (100g) low-fat yogurt   40
1oz (30g) low-fat cheese   73

23

Week 3 — yeast and alcohol

The third week of Stage II includes a variety of foods containing yeast, together with alcoholic drinks which also contain yeast.

At the Women's Nutritional Advisory Service, we find that sometimes yeast foods cause migraine headaches and abdominal symptoms or skin rashes. We have found that, often, when patients eliminate these foods from their diet, they feel well again and find it easier to lose weight.

This week we are asking you to reintroduce to your diet foods containing yeast, including:

- marmite and other yeast extracts
- vinegars
- mushrooms
- Oxo, Knorr and other stock cubes
- pickled foods
- condiments or sauces e.g. pickle or chutney

You will need to ensure you read the labels carefully when shopping, as many different types of food contain yeast or yeast extract.

Again, you may use the suggested menus as a guide, but regard the diet as flexible as long as:

- you include alcohol and yeast foods this week
- you keep within the confines of your daily calorie allowance.

Do remember to complete your daily chart if you experience any reactions, positive or negative.

If you like to drink alcohol regularly, you will probably find this is the most pleasant week of the diet, provided you don't experience a reaction to it. We trust you to be honest and note any adverse reaction on your chart!

One alcoholic drink is to be taken as half a pint of beer, one glass of wine, one small glass of sherry or one small measure of spirit.

Points to remember

- If you experience a reaction, immediately cut out the offending food or beverage.
- You will not be eating any grains or dairy produce this week apart from the permitted 2 slices of slimmer's

bread and 3floz (85ml) skimmed milk or low-fat yogurt.

- Please complete your weight and symptom charts on a daily basis so that you have all the information you require to complete the week-ending chart.

ELEANOR DODD

Since having her children five years previously Eleanor was unable to shift the stone (14lb/6.5kg) in weight she had gained. She had thrush 30 times in two years and experienced severe mood swings and bouts of anger. She and her husband were on the brink of breaking up and she could not cope with personal relationships.

'I was 11½ stone [160lb/73kg] when I began the WNAS diet. I had tried to diet many times before. I had been on low-calorie diets and diets out of newspapers, but I just could not stick to them. I could manage to lose five or six pounds and then I would break the diet, go back to normal food and put all the weight back on again.

'I used to feel so miserable dieting, always thinking about the foods I wanted but could not eat. I used to crave all sweet foods badly, and alcohol as well.

'I feel well again after following the WNAS programme. I no longer lash out at my husband and the children. In fact I feel happy to be alive and I am enjoying my relationship with my husband and my children. Plus I lost one stone in weight and this time I have not put the weight back on again.

'I felt fine on the WNAS diet. I felt that with the new knowledge I had gained about my diet I was eating sensibly, I no longer crave sweet foods, chocolate and alcohol and I feel that I'm physically on an even keel now.

'I found that cutting out dairy products has eased the feelings of irritability that I used to suffer from.

'I am definitely able to cope with things better now, especially the children. I have a new lease of life and will be forever indebted to the WNAS for their help and guidance.'

WEEK 3 — DAY 1

Breakfast	Calories
1oz (30g) cornflakes	104
3floz (85ml) skimmed milk	28

Mid-morning snack

4oz (115g) raw carrots	26

Lunch

5oz (140g) steamed haddock with a slice of lemon	138
2oz (55g) grilled mushrooms	7
4oz (115g) grilled tomatoes	16
1 alcoholic drink	60

Mid-afternoon snack

1 rice-cake with yeast extract	30

Dinner

*Tangy orange lamb	305
2oz (55g) brown rice	66
4oz (115g) carrots	21
4oz (115g) mangetout	27
1 alcoholic drink	60

Dessert

*Dried fruit compote	120
TOTAL CALORIES	**1,008**

FACTS

● For every £1 spent on food in the UK, 50p is spent on alcohol. On average, men consume three units of alcohol per day and women one unit per day. However, many of us are teetotal or are low drinkers.

● Yeast is used primarily in the baking and brewing industries. It is like a digestive aid breaking down some foods, such as wheat, into more digestible and more edible forms.

Daily chart

Today's weight _____

Symptoms _____

_____

_____

_____

_____

WEEK 3 — DAY 2

Breakfast	Calories
1oz (30g) Rice Krispies	105
3floz (85ml) skimmed milk	28

Mid-morning snack

4oz (115g) raw carrots	26

Lunch

4oz (115g) smoked mackerel	280
*Bean and sweetcorn salad	25

Mid-afternoon snack

1 tablespoon of raisins	20
1 alcoholic drink	60

Dinner

4oz (115g) grilled chicken breast	140
*Cider and red cabbage	145
4oz (115g) broccoli	20
1 glass of wine	60

Dessert

*Baked apple, stuffed with 1 tablespoon raisins	100

TOTAL CALORIES	1,009

FACTS

● In the last 40 years, total alcohol consumption has doubled. The main increase has been in wine and spirits with a small fall in beer. On average, 6 per cent of our daily calorie intake comes from alcoholic beverages. In alcoholics this can be as much as 50 per cent.

● Baker's yeast breaks down some of the indigestible phytic acid in wheat and generates carbon dioxide in the process, causing the bread to rise. This makes it easier for us to digest the wheat.

Daily chart

Today's weight _____

Symptoms _____

_____

_____

_____

_____

WEEK 3 — DAY 3

Breakfast	Calories
1 scrambled egg	80
2 medium tomatoes, grilled	16
2oz (55g) grilled mushrooms	7

Mid-morning snack

1 tablespoon raisins	20

Lunch

*Sea salad	205
2oz (55g) brown rice	66

Mid-afternoon snack

4oz (115g) raw carrot	26
1 alcoholic drink	60

Dinner

*Trout in cider	210
4oz (115g) boiled potatoes	90
4oz (115g) French beans	8
4oz (115g) cauliflower	10
1 alcoholic drink	60

Dessert

*Pancakes with lemon and sugar	150

TOTAL CALORIES	1,008

FACTS

● Most alcoholic drinks, like sugar, are empty calories, as they do not provide any significant amount of protein, vitamins or minerals. Small amounts of vitamins and minerals in beer are more than offset by the adverse effect of alcohol on your nutritional state. Alcohol in conjunction with sugar increases the release of insulin, a hormone which may cause a lowering of blood sugar and may lead to obesity.

● Brewer's yeast is used to turn sugar into alcohol — a process that also generates carbon dioxide which puts the fizz in Champagne.

Daily chart

Today's weight _____

Symptoms _____

_____

_____

_____

_____

WEEK 3 — DAY 4

Breakfast	Calories
1oz (30g) Rice Krispies	105
3floz (85ml) skimmed milk	28

Mid-morning snack

1 tablespoon raisins	20

Lunch

Weight Watchers mushroom soup	70
1 slice of slimmer's bread	40
*Beetroot and cabbage salad	47
2oz (55g) butter beans	52
1 alcoholic drink	60

Mid-afternoon snack

1oz (30g) dried apricots	51

Dinner

4oz (115g) grilled lamb chop	222
3 tablespoons (45ml) gravy with Oxo, Bovril and mint sauce	11
4oz (115g) cauliflower	10
4oz (115g) boiled potatoes	90
4oz (115g) marrow	8
1 glass of alcohol	60

Dessert

*Grape and white wine jelly	135
TOTAL CALORIES	**1,009**

FACTS

● The effect of alcohol on nutrients is particularly powerful against vitamin B, magnesium and zinc. Not only does alcohol displace essential nutrients from the diet, but it blocks their absorption by the body.

● Alcoholic drinks have a significant calorie content, ranging from about 50 calories for a small measure of spirit to 70–130 for a glass of wine and 90–130 for half a pint of beer. Excess alcohol consumption is associated with premature death, and some 1,100 people are killed on the road in the UK each year as a result of drunken driving.

Daily chart

Today's weight _____

Symptoms _____

_____

_____

_____

_____

_____

WEEK 3 — DAY 5

Breakfast	**Calories**
4oz (115g) mushrooms poached in water	14
1 slice of slimmer's bread	40
1 teaspoon (5ml) low-calorie spread	25

Mid-morning snack

1 tablespoon of raisins	20
2oz (55g) raw carrot	13

Lunch

*Stir-fried chicken and vegetables	242
2oz (55g) brown rice	66
1 glass of alcohol	60

Mid-afternoon snack

1oz (30g) dried apricots	51

Dinner

*Haddock kedgeree (smoked)	290
*Green salad with 2oz (55g) raw mushrooms	39
1 glass of alcohol	60

Dessert

*Grapefruit sorbet	85

TOTAL CALORIES	**1,005**

FACTS

● Alcohol is toxic to the ovaries and the testes. Levels of oestrogen in women and testosterone in men are reduced by heavy drinking. In men this results in loss of libido and reduces sperm formation and size of the testes. In women it results in irregular, heavy or even absent periods. Ovaries, breasts and external genitalia are reduced in size, and vaginal secretions reduced.

● Some people can be quite sensitive or allergic to baker's or brewer's yeast and this can cause skin reactions, including urticaria (nettle-rash) and eczema, and sometimes bowel problems.

Daily chart

Today's weight _____

Symptoms _____

_____

_____

_____

_____

WEEK 3 — DAY 6

Breakfast	Calories
2 pieces of fresh fruit chopped with 3½oz (100g) Shape yogurt	140
1 tablespoon raisins	20

Mid-morning snack

4oz (115g) raw carrots	26
3oz (85g) stick of celery	6

Lunch

Weight Watchers beef and vegetable soup	70
*Beansprout salad	65
Jacket potato	96
1 teaspoon (5ml) low-calorie spread	25
1 alcoholic drink	60

Mid-afternoon snack

1oz (30g) dried apricots	51

Dinner

*Sherried prawns	160
4oz (115g) broccoli	20
4oz (115g) mangetout	20
2oz (55g) brown rice	66
1 alcoholic drink	60

Dessert

*Brandied apricot flambé	115
TOTAL CALORIES	**1,000**

FACTS

● Alcohol can cause low blood sugar (hypoglycaemia), usually 6–36 hours after a binge; it is worsened by not eating food.

● Ten per cent of alcoholics develop liver disease. The rest often develop high blood pressure, heart disease, kidney or brain damage, strokes, peptic ulcers, obesity, loss of libido, infertility, and mental illness.

● Yeast extract e.g. marmite, some wines, vinegar and also cheese are all very rich in certain chemicals called amines, which can trigger off a migraine headache in sensitive people.

Daily chart

Today's weight _____

Symptoms _____

_____

_____

_____

_____

_____

WEEK 3 — DAY 7

Breakfast	Calories
*Dried fruit compote	120
3½oz (100g) Shape yogurt	40

Mid-morning snack

4oz (115g) raw carrots	26

Lunch

4oz (115g) sardines in tomato sauce mixed with 1 tablespoon vinegar	200
*Beetroot and cabbage salad	47
2oz (55g) brown rice	66
1 alcoholic drink	60

Mid-afternoon snack

1 fresh orange	50

Dinner

4oz (115g) roast beef (topside)	176
3 tablespoons (45ml) gravy with Oxo cube	11
4oz (115g) marrow	8
4oz (115g) spring greens	11
4oz (115g) boiled potatoes	90
1 alcoholic drink	60

Dessert

*Rhubarb and ginger mousse	50
TOTAL CALORIES	**1,015**

FACTS

● Women consuming one unit of alcohol per day at the time of conception and during pregnancy have babies that are smaller and thus at greater risk of illness.

● Foods rich in yeast include all bread except soda bread, all yeast extract spreads e.g. marmite, many savoury snacks, alcoholic beverages, vinegar and foods preserved in or containing vinegar.

Daily chart

Today's weight _____

Symptoms _____

_____

_____

_____

_____

_____

WEEK-ENDING CHART Stage II				
Date				
Total weight loss this week	Suspect foods discovered	Safe foods discovered	General degree of well-being*	Any other comments or observations
Weight at beginning of week				
Weight at end of week				
Change in weight				

*Score degree of well-being
Very well 3   Well 2   Fair 1   Unwell 0

REVIEW YOUR PROGRESS

If foods containing yeast and alcohol were a surprise to you, i.e. you had to cut some of them out of your diet, don't feel too disappointed. Be encouraged by the fact that you will be feeling healthier and lighter by the end of the diet.

If the yeast foods caused you to have an abdominal reaction, then you may find the weight loss came to a standstill this week. Do not be too concerned as you will find you lose the extra weight once you have eliminated the offending foods again.

Make sure you complete your week-ending chart accurately, and remember:

- to record your weight loss for the week
- to record all details about any foods or drinks that may have caused symptoms or weight gain
- that you will not be drinking alcohol or eating foods that contain yeast next week — which is the final week of Stage II.

RECIPES

Tangy orange lamb

Serves 4   Calories per serving 305

8 × 5oz (140g) escalopes of lamb
¼ pint (140ml) pure orange juice
4 tablespoons (60ml) white wine
2 tablespoons ground ginger
2 onions, sliced
1 tablespoon sultanas
1 orange, peeled and broken into
  segments

1. Place the lamb in a casserole dish.
2. Mix orange juice, wine, and ginger together and pour over lamb. Leave to marinade for 45 minutes.
3. Gently fry the onion for 1 minute, add the lamb and fry on both sides. Then add the marinade and simmer for 8–10 minutes.
4. Add the orange and sultanas, and simmer for a further 2 minutes. Add 1–2 tablespoons of orange juice if necessary.
5. Serve immediately.

Sea salad

Serves 4   Calories per serving 205

8oz (225g) squid, sliced thinly
1lb (455g) mussels, cooked
4oz (115g) peeled prawns
2 tomatoes, sliced
1 small onion, chopped finely
1 clove of garlic, crushed
1 tablespoon white wine vinegar
1 tablespoon chopped parsley
1 tablespoon (15ml) lemon juice
2 tablespoons (30ml) white wine
Pepper to taste

1. Cook the squid in a pan of boiling water for 2–3 minutes, remove and leave to drain.
2. Mix together all the ingredients and chill in fridge before serving.

Cider and red cabbage

Serves 6   Calories per serving 145

1lb (455g) red cabbage, shredded
½ pint (285ml) cider
2 tablespoons (30ml) lemon juice
2 tablespoons chopped mixed herbs
2oz (55g) sultanas
2 medium courgettes, sliced
2 teaspoons sunflower oil
2 onions, sliced
2 apples, cored and chopped
8oz (225g) leeks, chopped
8oz (225g) potatoes, part-baked and
    sliced
Freshly ground black pepper
2 teaspoons chives
1 teaspoon low-fat spread

1. Brush a non-stick pan with oil, add the onion and the chopped leeks, and fry for 1–2 minutes. Add the cabbage and cook for another 6 minutes.
2. Add the cider, lemon juice, herbs and sultanas and cook for 10 minutes, stirring occasionally.
3. Add the courgette, apple and pepper, and cook for a further 2 minutes.
4. Transfer to an oven-proof dish, cover with potatoes and dot with low-fat spread.
5. Cover and cook for 35–40 minutes at 190°C/375°F/Gas Mark 5.
6. Brown potatoes under grill, and sprinkle with chives to serve.

Trout in cider

Serves 2   Calories per serving 210

2 × 5–6oz (140–170g) trout, gutted
2 small dessert apples, peeled and
    chopped
1 small onion, chopped
½ pint (285ml) dry cider
2 lemon slices to decorate
1 tablespoon parsley, finely chopped

1. Mix apple and chopped onion together with the parsley, and stuff into each trout.
2. Place the fish in an oven-proof dish. Pour on the cider and season with pepper.
3. Cover and cook in the oven (190°C/375°F/Gas Mark 5) for 30–40 minutes.
4. Serve with 2 tablespoons of the liquid and a slice of lemon to garnish.

Stir-fry chicken and vegetables

Serves 1   Calories 242

4oz (115g) chicken breast, cut into strips
4oz (115g) mushrooms, thickly sliced
2oz (55g) courgettes, sliced
2oz (55g) French beans
2 tablespoons oil
1 pinch of nutmeg
Freshly ground black pepper

1. Heat the oil in a large saucepan or wok.
2. Add the chicken and stir-fry for 3 minutes.
3. Add the vegetables and nutmeg.
4. Stir-fry for a further 5–8 minutes before serving.

Sherried prawns

Serves 2   Calories per serving 160

6oz (170g) peeled prawns
1 green pepper, seeded and cut into matchstick strips
4oz (115g) water chestnuts (canned)
4 tablespoons (60ml) sherry
1 tablespoon (15ml) lemon juice
1 teaspoon of finely-chopped root ginger
1 tablespoon chopped spring onions
3oz (85g) beansprouts
Freshly ground black pepper
1 teaspoon oil

1. Soak the prawns in a mixture of the sherry, lemon juice and ginger for at least 1 hour.
2. Heat the oil, add the spring onions and stir-fry for 1–2 minutes.
3. Add the prawn mixture, beansprouts, water chestnuts, and green pepper.
4. Stir over a moderate heat for 4–5 minutes.
5. Season with pepper and serve.

NB: **Haddock Kedgeree** — see Stage II, Week 2 for recipe, but use smoked haddock in Week 3. For salad recipes see Stage I.

Dried fruit compote

Serves 2   Calories per serving 120

4oz (115g) mixture of dried fruits,
  e.g. peaches, prunes, apples,
  apricots and pears
4floz (115ml) orange juice
2 whole cloves
2-inch (5cm) stick of cinnamon
Zest and juice of ½ lemon

1. Wash the fruit and place in a
   bowl with the orange juice,
   spices, lemon juice and zest.
2. Leave to soak overnight.
3. Next day, if the juice has been
   absorbed, add 2 tablespoons of
   water. Then place mixture in a
   saucepan and bring to the boil,
   cover and simmer on a very low
   heat for 10–15 minutes.
4. Transfer to a serving bowl,
   removing cinnamon and cloves.
   Leave to cool or serve warm.

Grape and white wine jelly

Serves 4   Calories per serving 135

8oz (225g) green grapes, skinned,
  halved and seeded
½ pint (285ml) diluted apple juice
½ pint (285ml) dry white wine
4 teaspoons powdered gelatine
Green grapes to decorate

1. Place the gelatine and three
   tablespoons of apple juice in a
   small bowl, stand the bowl in a
   saucepan of hot water and stir
   over a gentle heat until dissolved.
2. Combine the remaining apple
   juice and white wine with the
   gelatine mixture and put to one
   side until syrupy.
3. Stir the prepared grapes into the
   jelly.
4. Pour into 1½ pint (30floz/850ml)
   jelly mould or 4 individual
   moulds.
5. Chill for approximately 2–3
   hours until set.
6. Carefully turn out the jelly onto
   a serving plate and decorate with
   the extra grapes.

Brandied apricot flambé

Serves 2   Calories per serving 115

8 apricots, halved and stoned
6 tablespoons (90ml) water
4 tablespoons caster sugar
2 tablespoons (30ml) brandy
1 teaspoon arrowroot

1. Place the halved apricots and water in a saucepan and heat gently.
2. As the apricots soften, sprinkle sugar over them, cover and simmer on a very low heat until cooked but still hard.
3. Strain the apricots (saving the juice) and place in an oven-proof dish.
4. Mix the arrowroot with a little syrup from the paste and then mix with the remaining syrup and return to the heat.
5. Bring to the boil, stirring constantly.
6. Pour the thickened syrup over the apricots.
7. Heat the apricots and syrup over a low heat while warming the brandy.
8. Remove the apricots from the heat, gently pour on the brandy, and ignite.

NB: **Rhubarb and ginger mousse** and **Baked apple** — see Stage I; **Gooseberry mousse** and **Grapefruit sorbet** — see Stage II, Week 2.

PACKED LUNCHES

You can use any of the packed lunches from Stage I, but do try to add some yeasty or pickled foods and vinegar dressings.

	Calories
Fruity cabbage, or any other salad, with 2oz (55g) raw mushrooms, plus two pickled onions	78

You can add any of the following to these salads:

	Calories
4oz (115g) smoked haddock	114
4oz (115g) smoked mackerel	280
2 rice-cakes with marmite	60

SNACKS

1 teaspoon marmite spread	2
1 tablespoon raisins	20
1oz (30g) dried apricots	51

24

Week 4 — tea, coffee, chocolate and cola

Having eliminated some traditional habits such as drinking tea, coffee, and cola-based drinks, and eating chocolate for seven weeks, you now have the chance to include these in your diet once again.

Before getting too excited, you must remember that this is a weight-loss diet and consequently drinks and foods containing chocolate must be included in the diet within the confines of your calorie allowance, and that doesn't mean just eating 1,000 calories worth of chocolate per day (equal to 2½ king-size Mars Bars).

ALLOWANCES

The daily allowances for this week are as follows:

Tea	up to 6 cups per day
Coffee	up to 6 cups per day
Cola*	1–2 cans per day
Chocolate	1×2oz (55g) bar of chocolate per day

*Not caffeine-free, but low-calorie.

This week you can drink your tea and coffee with milk if you would prefer.

Bear in mind that 1floz (30ml) of skimmed milk has 5 calories.

SIDE-EFFECTS

The reactions you may experience to these drinks and chocolate, having cleansed your system of them or more importantly having overcome any addiction you may have had, may include:

- migraine headache
- irritability
- depression
- anxiety
- shaky nervous feeling
- increased passage of urine
- mental overactivity
- insomnia
- weight gain.

There are suggested menus for each day as for the previous weeks, with the key facts, and daily charts to complete. By now you will have become an old hand at completing charts, logging your daily weight, and entering any adverse reactions and symptoms you may have experienced.

SALLY CLARK

Sally had been two stones (28lb/12.5kg) overweight for ten years following the birth of her son. She was always looking for quick weight-loss diets. She tried low-calorie diets for a few weeks.

'I tried the Univite diet and any other diet from a women's magazine that I came across. I did lose weight but found that the weight returned as soon as I returned to my normal diet. Whilst dieting I felt that my attempts were always too drastic. I didn't have the correct nourishment. I used to skip breakfast, and as a result felt unwell. I was always looking for a short-term miracle.

'I felt so unwell. I was awful, mentally, to my husband and my son. I realized I had to do something about it myself.

'I began the WNAS diet. It took me four to five months to get back to the weight I was before I was pregnant. I lost two stones in all. I lost about 1–1¼lb [455–570g] per week steadily after the initial weight loss on the WNAS diet. I felt much better on the diet. I no longer had cravings for sweet or spicy food. I was calmer, nicer to my family and much more like my old self. I found that caffeine in coffee was contributing to my feelings of nervous tension. As soon as I cut out brown bread my stomach cramps went, and all my unpleasant bowel-related symptoms went also, as well as my headaches, sore tongue and dandruff.

'I feel far more contented and in control now. The WNAS diet has taught me which foods suit me most.

'I have much more energy. I walk two miles a day and I have taken up gardening again.'

You are welcome to vary the diet, but do make sure you eat other foods besides chocolate this week!

POINTS TO REMEMBER

Once again, just to refresh your memory:

- If you experience any signs or symptoms that indicate you may be allergic to a food or drink, eliminate it from your diet quickly.
- You will not be consuming any grains, dairy products, yeast, or alcohol this week.
- Please complete your daily charts so that you have an accurate running record. From this you can record the information required on the week-ending chart. You will also be able to do the *grand progress review* (page 227).

WEEK 4 — DAY 1

Breakfast	Calories
1oz (30g) Rice Krispies	105
3floz (85ml) skimmed milk	28
1 chopped apple	50
2 cups of tea or coffee	10

Mid-morning snack

4oz (115g) raw carrots	26
1 cup of tea or coffee	5

Lunch

*Spinach and sweetcorn omelette	200
*Green salad	32
1 can of cola (low-calorie)	1

Mid-afternoon snack

1 piece of fresh fruit	50
1 cup of tea or coffee	5

Dinner

*Seafood kebab	120
2oz (55g) brown rice	66
*Vegetable salad	50

Dessert

2oz (55g) chocolate	260
2 cups of tea or coffee	10

TOTAL CALORIES	1,018

FACTS

● Tea and coffee are the most popular beverages in the UK. On average, British adults consume four cups of tea and two cups of coffee per day. Tea and coffee both contain appreciable amounts of caffeine, a drug with stimulant properties. Our average intake of caffeine from tea and coffee is around 500 milligrams (mg) per day, enough to produce a significant effect.

● Smaller but still significant amounts of caffeine may be found in cola-based drinks, some pain-killing preparations, and in chocolate.

Daily chart

Today's weight _____

Symptoms _____

_____

_____

_____

_____

_____

WEEK 4 — DAY 2

Breakfast	**Calories**
1 boiled egg (size 3)	80
1 slice of slimmer's bread	40
2 cups of tea or coffee	10

Mid-morning snack

4oz (115g) raw carrots	26
1 cup of tea or coffee	5

Lunch

Jacket potato	96
4oz (115g) Weight Watchers baked beans	61
1 cup of tea or coffee	5

Mid-afternoon snack

2oz (55g) chocolate	260
1 cola (low-calorie)	1
1 rice-cake	28
1 teaspoon low-calorie jam	10

Dinner

Lean Cuisine chicken and oriental vegetables	259

Dessert

*Chocolate fruit roll	120
1 cup of tea or coffee	5

TOTAL CALORIES	1,006

FACTS

● A cup of black tea or black coffee contains no calories, but a cup of white tea or coffee with 2 teaspoons of sugar can provide up to 60 calories — and with an average of 6 cups per day, that could be 360 calories per day!

● The tannin in tea and coffee inhibits the absorption of iron and zinc from the diet. This effect is particularly on iron from vegetable, non-meat sources, so that the tea-drinking vegetarian may be particularly at risk.

Daily chart

Today's weight _____

Symptoms _____

_____

_____

_____

_____

_____

WEEK 4 — DAY 3

Breakfast	Calories
2 pieces of chopped fruit	100
3½oz (100g) Shape yogurt	40
1 cup of tea or coffee	5

Mid-morning snack

3oz (85g) stick of celery	6
1 tea or coffee	5

Lunch

2oz (55g) brown rice	66
*Bean salad	110
2oz (55g) lettuce	7
1 medium tomato	
(2oz/55g)	8
2 cups of tea or coffee	10

Mid-afternoon snack

1 cola (low-calorie)	1
4oz (115g) raw carrot	26

Dinner

*Chicken with prawn sauce	250
4oz (115g) boiled potatoes	90
4oz (115g) marrow	8
4oz (115g) French beans	8

Dessert

2oz (55g) chocolate	260
2 cups of tea or coffee	10
TOTAL CALORIES	**1,010**

FACTS

● Caffeine, at a dosage of 200–250mg (approximately half our average daily intake) can be mildly stimulating, elevating mood and improving concentration. Larger doses produce symptoms like those of anxiety or nervousness — increased passage of urine, insomnia, withdrawal headache, diarrhoea, anxiety, rapid heart-beat and tremors.

● At higher doses, caffeine is truly a drug of addiction. Withdrawal produces emotional changes, immobility, lethargy, and headaches which can be severe. These symptoms are usually worse in the first few days, lessening thereafter.

Daily chart

Today's weight _____

Symptoms _____

_____

_____

_____

_____

WEEK 4 — DAY 4

Breakfast	Calories
1oz (30g) cornflakes	104
3floz (85ml) skimmed milk	28
2 cups of tea or coffee	10

Mid-morning snack

4oz (115g) raw carrot	26
1 cola (low-calorie)	1
1 cup of tea or coffee	5

Lunch

4oz (115g) Weight Watchers baked beans	61
Jacket potato	96
*Courgette and cauliflower salad	27

Mid-afternoon snack

1 cup of tea or coffee	5
2oz (55g) chocolate	260
6oz (170g) sticks of celery	12

Dinner

*Haddock Florentine	170
4oz (115g) boiled potatoes	90
4oz (115g) mangetout	27
4oz (115g) French beans	8
2 cups of tea or coffee	10

Dessert

*Rhubarb and ginger mousse	50
TOTAL CALORIES	**990**

FACTS

● Those with a nervous disposition and who are anxious or panicky are more likely to be sensitive to the adverse effects of caffeine. It is these people who should avoid it.

● Insomnia can be easily caused by caffeine from tea and coffee, especially when either are consumed in the evening. Caffeine delays the onset of sleep, keeping you wide awake until the small hours. Again, the effect varies a lot from individual to individual.

Daily chart

Today's weight _____

Symptoms _____

_____

_____

_____

_____

WEEK 4 — DAY 5

Breakfast	Calories
2 fresh fruits, chopped	100
3½oz (100g) Shape yogurt	40
1 cup of tea or coffee	5

Mid-morning snack

2oz (55g) raw carrot	13
2 cups of tea or coffee	10

Lunch

4oz (115g) tinned pilchards (in tomato sauce)	144
*Green salad	32
1 slice of slimmer's bread	40
1 teaspoon (5ml) low-calorie spread	25
1 can of cola (low-calorie)	1

Mid-afternoon snack

2 cups of tea or coffee	10
2oz (55g) chocolate	260

Dinner

Lean Cuisine beef julienne	245

Dessert

1 cup of tea or coffee	5
*Jellied grapefruit	70

TOTAL CALORIES	1,000

FACTS

● Caffeine has stimulant effects on the heart and may cause a mild increase in blood pressure or heart rate. Palpitations — irregular or rapid heart rate — can be caused by excess tea or coffee in susceptible individuals.

● Caffeine may cause a rise in blood sugar and this, by stimulating insulin release, may lead to fat deposition. Even decaffeinated coffee may stimulate acid production by the stomach and then predispose you to indigestion, heartburn and peptic ulcers.

Daily chart

Today's weight _____

Symptoms _____

_____

_____

_____

_____

WEEK 4 — DAY 6

Breakfast	Calories
1 boiled egg (size 3)	80
1 slice of slimmer's bread	40
2 cups of tea or coffee	10

Mid-morning snack

2oz (55g) chocolate	260
1 cup of tea or coffee	5

Lunch

*Orange and carrot soup	55
2 rice-cakes or 1 slice of slimmer's bread	56

Mid-afternoon snack

4oz (115g) raw carrot	26
1 can of cola (low-calorie)	1
1 cup of tea or coffee	5

Dinner

*Turkey in lemon sauce	320
2oz (55g) brown rice	66
*Tomato and celery salad	20

Dessert

*Cranberry sorbet	50
2 cups of tea or coffee	10

TOTAL CALORIES	1,004

FACTS

● Large amounts of coffee (and possibly tea) interfere with the absorption of magnesium. This mineral is important in the health of the nervous system and often deficient in women with pre-menstrual syndrome.

● Tea in large doses can have adverse effect on vitamin B_1 (thiamine) also very important for the nervous system.

Daily chart

Today's weight _____

Symptoms _____

_____

_____

_____

_____

WEEK 4 — DAY 7

Breakfast	Calories
½ grated apple	25
3½oz (100g) Shape yogurt	40
2 cups of tea or coffee	10

Mid-morning snack

3oz (85g) stick of celery	6
2 cups of tea or coffee	10

Lunch

*Chicken and pineapple kebab	230
*Root salad	31

Mid-afternoon snack

2oz (55g) chocolate	260
1 can of low-calorie cola	1

Dinner

4oz (115g) roast lamb	196
4oz (115g) potatoes	90
4oz (115g) carrots	21
4oz (115g) cabbage	10

Dessert

*Rhubarb and ginger mousse	50
2 cups of tea or coffee	10
TOTAL CALORIES	**990**

FACTS

● Chocolate or chocolate liqueur is prepared by grinding the kernel of the cocoa bean and can be divided into two parts: the fatty part, cocoa butter, and the less fatty cocoa powder. Chocolate contains several active chemicals. It has small amounts of caffeine and related compounds called methyl xanthines, and a further mood-stimulating substance, beta phenyl ethylamine.

● Chocolate and other forms of confectionery are the biggest source of hidden sugar in the average UK diet, comprising some 10 per cent of total sugar intake.

Daily chart

Today's weight _____

Symptoms _____

_____

_____

_____

_____

_____

REVIEW YOUR PROGRESS

Ideally, you will have come through this week and found that your liking for tea, coffee, chocolate and cola is now influenced by how much they like you.

While we firmly believe that 'a little of what you fancy does you good', you need to understand that none of the drinks or foods in this group are good, when taken in excess, for the human body. Quantities above six cups of tea or four cups of coffee per day provide enough caffeine to aggravate anxiety, depression and insomnia. Chocolate is best reserved as an occasional treat if you have weight-gain problems.

Once again this week you need to do the following, in preparation for the 'Grand Review':

- review your weight loss
- record any reactions you experienced
- make a note of any foods you have discarded
- note the positive drinks or foods that you have discovered.

WEEK-ENDING CHART
Stage II

Date

Total weight loss this week	Suspect foods discovered	Safe foods discovered	General degree of well-being*	Any other comments or observations
Weight at beginning of week				
Weight at end of week				
Change in weight				

*Score degree of well-being
Very well 3   Well 2   Fair 1   Unwell 0

RECIPES

Spinach and sweetcorn omelette

Serves 1   Calories 200

2 eggs (size 3)
2oz (55g) fresh/frozen spinach
1 tablespoon tinned sweetcorn
Freshly ground black pepper

1. Beat the eggs and add freshly ground black pepper.
2. Pour into a hot frying pan and leave to set for 1 minute.
3. Add the spinach and sweetcorn and leave for about a minute until heated.
4. Fold in half and serve.

Seafood kebab

Serves 4   Calories per serving 120

1lb (455g) cod fillet, skinned and cut into 1-inch (2.5cm) cubes
12 large prawns, peeled
4 firm tomatoes, quartered
1 small green pepper, seeded and cut into ¾-inch (2cm) pieces
2 tablespoons (30ml) fresh lemon juice
2 teaspoons finely chopped fresh basil *or* 1 teaspoon dried basil

1. Thread the cod, prawns, green pepper and tomatoes onto 8 skewers, and sprinkle with a little of the lemon juice and basil.
2. Cook under grill for 10 minutes, turning frequently and basting with the lemon juice.
3. When the cod is cooked, transfer to heated serving dish and serve.

Chicken with prawn sauce

Serves 6   Calories per serving 250

6 × 5oz (140g) chicken fillets
6oz (170g) peeled prawns
1 tablespoon (15ml) lemon juice
1 tablespoon (15ml) olive oil
3 green peppers, seeded and chopped
3 garlic cloves, peeled and chopped
3 fresh tomatoes, skinned and
chopped
2 sticks of celery, finely chopped

1. Place all the chopped vegetables into a casserole dish and sprinkle with freshly ground black pepper.
2. Place the chicken pieces on top and brush with a little of the oil.
3. Bake in the oven at 200°C/400°F/ Gas Mark 6 for 25–30 minutes. Remove fillets to a warm serving dish.
4. Heat the remaining oil and push the cooked vegetables through a sieve into the oil. Bring to the boil and add lemon juice and prawns. Cook for 3–4 minutes.
5. Spread the sauce over the chicken and serve.

Turkey in lemon sauce

Serves 4   Calories per serving 320

4 × 5oz (140g) skinned and boned
turkey breasts
Grated rind and juice of 1 lemon
1 small onion, finely chopped
1 tablespoon chopped fresh tarragon
2 tablespoons (30ml) olive oil
½ pint (285ml) chicken or vegetable
stock
2 teaspoons honey
Black pepper
2 teaspoons cornflour
1 tablespoon water

1. Heat the oil, fry the onion for 3–4 minutes. Add the turkey and lightly brown both sides.
2. Add the stock, honey, lemon rind and juice, and tarragon. Cover and simmer for 20 minutes.
3. Remove the turkey breasts and keep warm.
4. Blend cornflour and water to a smooth paste, remove pan with liquid in from the heat. Stir in the cornflour and return to heat to thicken.
5. Serve immediately.

Chicken and pineapple kebabs

Serves 2   Calories per serving 230

2×6oz (170g) chicken breasts
2 tablespoons (30ml) unsweetened
  pineapple juice
8oz (225g) pineapple, cut into 1-inch
  (2.5cm) cubes
1 courgette, thickly sliced
2 tablespoons (30ml) olive oil
1 tablespoon (15ml) lemon juice
1 garlic clove, crushed
Freshly ground black pepper
1 tablespoon freshly chopped mint

1. Mix olive oil, pineapple juice,
   lemon juice, garlic, chopped mint
   and fresh pepper.
2. Cover the chicken with the
   prepared marinade and leave for
   2–3 hours.
3. Thread 4 kebab skewers with
   chicken, pineapple and courgette.
   You should have 3 pieces of
   chicken on each skewer.
4. Cook under moderate heat,
   turning regularly and baste with
   marinade.
5. Serve hot.

NB: **Haddock Florentine** and **Orange and carrot soup** and salad recipes — see
Stage I.

Chocolate fruit roll

Makes 8 slices   Calories per serving 120

3 eggs (size 2)
1 tablespoon (15ml) concentrated
  apple juice to sweeten
½ teaspoon (2.5ml) sunflower oil
1½oz (45g) white self-raising flour
2 level tablespoons drinking
  chocolate powder
1 level tablespoon cocoa
2 tablespoons (30ml) hot water
8oz (225g) skimmed-milk cheese
4 level tablespoons strawberry jam
4oz (115g) fresh strawberries

1. Line a swiss roll tin (8×11 inch/
   20×28cm) with greaseproof
   paper, and brush with oil.
2. Separate the eggs, and whisk the
   yolks with the concentrated
   apple juice until light and creamy.
3. Sieve together the flour, drinking
   chocolate and cocoa.
4. Fold in the egg yolk mixture with
   the water.
5. Whisk the egg whites until stiff
   and then fold gently into the
   mixture.
6. Immediately turn into prepared
   tin and bake for 12–15 minutes at
   200°C/400°F/Gas Mark 6.
7. Turn out onto a greaseproof paper
   and cut off edges.
8. Roll up with the paper inside and
   leave to cool.
9. Unroll gently and spread with
   skimmed-milk cheese and jam,
   slice half the strawberries and
   place on the jam and then roll up
   again and place on serving dish.
   At this point slice one or two
   more strawberries and place on
   the top and arrange the rest of
   the strawberries around the edges
   to decorate.

NB: Recipes for **Jellied grapefruit**, **Cranberry sorbet** and **Rhubarb and ginger mousse** appear in Stage I.

PACKED LUNCHES
Choose from any of the Stage I packed lunches, page 151.

SNACKS
As Stage I (page 100), or:

1 cup of tea or coffee	5
1 can of low-calorie cola	1
2oz (55g) chocolate	260

25
Stage III — your long-term diet

THE GRAND PROGRESS REVIEW

You will need to set aside a bit of time to review the events of the last eight weeks. The simplest way to record your findings is to complete the chart on the next page. If you mark the details from your eight week-ending charts, this will give you easy reference to your records.

Complete the chart now.

YOUR FINDINGS

Once the chart is complete you will be able to see your findings at a glance. You will be able to see exactly which foods you felt well with and which foods you did not. Your next step is to become familiar with all the foods in the second column, Suspect foods, and to make a plan to avoid consuming these for the next few months.

Now you can move on to the final stage of the diet.

In this final stage of the diet we are looking to put together the best diet for your own metabolism and make-up, based on your findings. You will essentially be following the diet in Stage I, but adding to it any food or drink you now have listed in column 3 of the Grand Review Chart on page 228. You will need to work out a menu for yourself to follow, using the Stage I menus as a guide, but adding your own safe foods and drinks.

Follow your amended Stage I menu for the next two weeks, this time completing the charts on pages 230–231. Continue to weigh yourself daily and to mark your weight into the chart each day.

What should I do if I want to go on losing weight?

You should simply continue to follow your amended Stage I diet, which includes all the food from your 'safe' list, and keep your consumption down to around 1,000 calories per day. You can happily go on doing this until you reach your target weight. When that day arrives, you may follow the instructions in the next answer.

GRAND REVIEW CHART		
Weight loss	Suspect foods discovered	Safe foods discovered
Stage I:		
Week 1		
Week 2		
Week 3		
Week 4		
Stage II:		
Week 1		
Week 2		
Week 3		
Week 4		
Total lost		

What should I do when I have reached my target weight?

Simply increase your calorie consumption by up to 50 per cent. It is now recognized that people who have been on weight-reducing diets subsequently have a lower calorie requirement than they previously had. Do bear this in mind when increasing your volume of food. So, for example, if you previously ate 2,000 calories per day, you may now need to consume 1,500 to 1,800 instead, in order to maintain your new weight.

What if I get a reaction to a particular food after I have completed the diet?

If an adverse reaction to a food or drink occurs, you will recognize it! Now that you have the wealth of information about diet at your fingertips and the invaluable personal experience, you merely proceed in the same way as you did in Stage II of the diet.

For example, if you suddenly feel unwell after eating, either cut out the food you suspect for several weeks before trying it again, or if you are confused about which food or drink may be causing the problem, go back onto the Stage I diet for a week or so. If you are no longer on a weight-loss programme, don't forget to add more volume of food daily.

Long-term dieting

If you are dieting in the long term, you may need to take a multi-vitamin/multi-mineral supplement (e.g. Diet Balance) — if you need to be on a weight-loss programme for more than 10 weeks, or if you have to rely on prepared reduced-calorie meals, and especially if you have any of the signs suggestive of vitamin or mineral deficiency.

Should I follow the Stage III diet on a permanent basis?

The answer is simply 'yes'! Now that you have found the optimum diet for your own body — cherish it! Of course you can deviate occasionally, as long as you always come back to the diet as a routine.

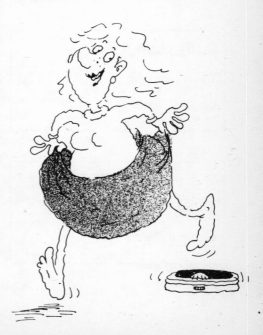

Stage III — Week 1

Daily chart 1

Today's weight _____

General degree
of well-being* _____

Daily chart 2

Today's weight _____

General degree
of well-being* _____

Daily chart 3

Today's weight _____

General degree
of well-being* _____

Daily chart 4

Today's weight _____

General degree
of well-being* _____

Daily chart 5

Today's weight _____

General degree
of well-being* _____

Daily chart 6

Today's weight _____

General degree
of well-being* _____

Daily chart 7

Today's weight _____

General degree
of well-being* _____

Week-ending chart

Date _____

Total weight loss
this week _____

General degree
of well-being* _____

Any other comments
or observations _____

*Score 0–3 as before

Stage III — Week 2

Daily chart 1

Today's weight _____

General degree
of well-being* _____

Daily chart 2

Today's weight _____

General degree
of well-being* _____

Daily chart 3

Today's weight _____

General degree
of well-being* _____

Daily chart 4

Today's weight _____

General degree
of well-being* _____

Daily chart 5

Today's weight _____

General degree
of well-being* _____

Daily chart 6

Today's weight _____

General degree
of well-being* _____

Daily chart 7

Today's weight _____

General degree
of well-being* _____

Week-ending chart

Date _____

Total weight loss
this week _____

General degree
of well-being* _____

Any other comments
or observations _____

*Score 0–3 as before

Appendix 1
Suggested reading list

RECIPE BOOKS

The Allergy Cook Book, Danila Armstrong, SRD and Dr Andrew Cant. Octopus Books, London. 1986. (Especially of value in Stage I of the diet.)

The Make It Simple Cook Book, Weight Watchers Step by Step Guide to Easy Cooking, Anne Page-Wood. New English Library, Sevenoaks, England. 1989.

The Slimmers' Year, Anne Ager, Julie Hamilton, Miriam Palunin. Hamlyn, London. 1989.

Seasonal Salads, David Scott and Paddy Byrne. Ebury Press, London. 1985.

Salads, Mary Cadogen. Sainsbury's Recipe Library. 1986.

Calorie Counted Meals, Alex Barber, Sainsbury's Recipe Library. 1986.

Raw Energy Recipes, Leslie and Susannah Kenton, Century, London. 1985.

HEALTH

Nutritional Medicine, Dr Stephen Davies and Dr Alan Stewart, Pan, London. 1987.

The Food Scandal, Caroline Walker and Geoffrey Cannon, Century, London. 1986.

Beat PMT Through Diet, Maryon Stewart with contributions from Dr Guy Abraham and Dr Alan Stewart, Ebury Press, London. 1987.

Candida Albicans — Could Yeast Be Your Problem? Leon Chaitow, Thorsons, Wellingborough. 1985.

Candida — Diet Against It, Luc de Schepper, Foulsham, Slough. 1989.

Candida Albicans Yeast Free Cookbook, Pat Connolly and Associates of the Price Pattenger Nutrition Foundation, Keats Pub. Inc. 1986.

MEDICAL

Manual of Nutrition. 8th edition. Ministry of Agriculture, Fisheries and Food. Her Majesty's Stationery Office, London. 1981.

Smoking or Health. Third Report. Royal College of Physicians of London. Pitman Publishing Ltd, London. 1979.

Tomorrow I'll Be Slim: The Psychology of Dieting. Sara Gilbert. Routledge, London. 1989.

Food Allergy. Patricia Scowen. B. Edsal & Co. Ltd, London. 1985.

Pure, White and Deadly. John Yudkin. Viking (Penguin Books Ltd), London. 1986.

The Food Intolerance Diet Book. Elizabeth Workman, SRD, Dr Virginia Alun Jones, Dr John Hunter. Martin Dunitz Ltd, London. 1986.

Clinical Nutrition, Student Reviews, Graham Neale, MA, BSc, MB, ChB, FRCP. Heinemann Medical Books, London. 1988.

Handbook of Dietary Fibre. Mark L. Dreher. Marcel Dekker, Inc., New York. 1987.

Treat Obesity Seriously. J. S. Garrow, MD, PhD, FRCP. Churchill Livingstone, London. 1981.

Human Nutrition and Dietetics. R. Passmore, M. A. Eastwood. 8th edition. Churchill Livingstone, London. 1986.

Manual of Dietetic Practice. Briony Thomas (ed). Blackwell Scientific Publications, Oxford. 1988.

Appendix 2
Nutritional supplements

UK

Diet Balance — available from leading chemists and other health food shops.

Health Insurance Plus — available mail order from Nature's Best, 1 Lamberts Road, PO Box 1, Tunbridge Wells, TN2 3EQ.

Optivite — available from Holland & Barrett, Boots, independent chemists and health food shops.

Sugar Factor — available by mail order from Nature's Best, address as above.

Cantamega 2000 — available from health food shops.

Quest Once-a-Day — available from health food shops.

AUSTRALIA

Diet Balance — available through Blackmores Laboratories.

P.M.T. — available through Blackmores Laboratories.

Sugar Factor — available through Blackmores Laboratories.

USA

Optivite — available from Optimox US, 2720 Monterey Street, Suite 4, Torrance, CA 90503, United States.

Appendix 3
Useful addresses

NB: Please note that London codes will change from 6 May 1990. If you have difficulty obtaining the correct number after that date, there is a free enquiry number: 0800 800 873.

Alcoholics Anonymous (AA), General Services Office, PO Box 1, Stonebow House, Stonebow, York YO1 2NJ. Tel: (0904) 644026

Anorexia and Bulimia Nervosa Association, Tottenham Woman's and Health Centre, Annexe C, Tottenham Town Hall, Town Hall Approach, London N15 4RX. Tel: (01) 885 3936 Wednesday 6–9pm

Asset, The National Association for Health and Exercise Teachers, 202 The Avenue, Kennington, Oxford OX1 5RN. Tel: (0865) 736066

Clear (Campaign for Lead-free Air), 3 Endsleigh Street, London WC1H 0DD. Tel: (01) 278 9686

College Of Health, 18 Victoria Park Square, Bethnal Green, London E2 9PF. Tel: (01) 980 6263

Friends Of The Earth Ltd, 26–28 Underwood Street, London N1 7JQ. Tel: (01) 490 1555

National Society for Research into Allergy, PO Box 45, Hinckley, Leicestershire LE10 1JY.

Samaritans, 17 Uxbridge Road, Slough SL1 1SN. Tel: (0753) 327133

The Henry Doubleday Research Association, Ryton Gardens, National Centre For Organic Gardening, Ryton-on-Dunsmore, Coventry CV8 3LG. Tel: (0203) 303517

The Soil Association, 86–88 Colston Street, Bristol BS1 5BB. Tel: (0272) 290661

Tranx (Tranquillizer Recovery & New Existence), Ms Joan Gerome, 17 Peel Road, Wealdstone, Middlesex. Tel: (01) 427 2065

Tranx Release (Northampton), Anita Gordon, 24 Hazelwood Road, Northampton NN1 1LN. Tel: (0604) 250976

Women's Nutritional Advisory Service, PO Box 268, Hove, East Sussex BN3 1RW. Tel: (0273) 771336

Findus Foods, St Georges House, Park Lane, Croydon, Surrey, CR9 1NR. Tel: (01) 686 3333

Heinz, Hayes Park, Hayes, Middlesex, UB4 8AL. Tel: (01) 573 7757

St Ivels Ltd, Dorkham House, Eldene Drive, Swindon, Wiltshire SN3 3TU. Tel: (0793) 488333

AUSTRALIA

Adelaide Women's Health Advisory Service, 64 Pennington Terrace, Nth Adelaide SA 5006. Tel: (08) 267 5366

Brisbane Women's Community Health, PO Box 248, Woolloongabba QLD 4102. Tel: (07) 393 9974

Liverpool Women's Health Centre, 26 Bathurst Street, Liverpool NSW 2170. Tel: (02) 601 3555

Melbourne Women's Health Resource Collective, 653 Nicholson Street, Nth Carlton, VIC 3054. Tel: (03) 380 9974

Perth Women's Health Care House, 100 Aberdeen Street, Northbridge, WA 6000. Tel: (09) 227 8122

Women's Health Advisory Service, 187 Glenmore Road, Paddington, NSW 2021. Tel: (02) 331 1294

NEW ZEALAND

Gisborne Women's Centre, 1st Floor, Old National Bank Bldg, Gladstone Road, PO Box 1398, Gisborne. Tel: 76 247

New Plymouth Women's Centre, PO Box 4030, New Plymouth. Tel: 84 957

Papakura Women's Centre, 4 Opaneke Road, Papkura, Auckland. Tel: 2999 466

Tauranga Women's Centre, PO Box 368, Tauranga. Tel: 83 530

West Auckland Women's Centre, 111 McLeod Road, Te Atatu, Auckland. Tel: 8366 381

Whakatane Women's Centre, PO Box 3049, Ohope. Tel: 076 24757

Women's Health Collective, 63 Ponsonby Road, Auckland. Tel: 764 506

Women's Health Collective, PO Box 4253, 51 Walde Grove, Palmerston North. Tel: 70 314 (10am–9pm)

USA AND CANADA

The American Academy of Environmental Medicine, PO Box 16106, Denver, Colorado 80216. Tel: (303) 622 9755

Index

Index to recipes